THE SLEEP APNEA SYNDROME, MORE AS AN ILLNESS

THE SLEEP APNEA SYNDROME, MORE AS AN ILLNESS

A. BUTTNER

Nova Science Publishers, Inc.
New York

For permission to use material from this book please contact us:
Telephone 631-231-7269; Fax 631-231-8175
Web Site: http://www.novapublishers.com

NOTICE TO THE READER

The Publisher has taken reasonable care in the preparation of this book, but makes no expressed or implied warranty of any kind and assumes no responsibility for any errors or omissions. No liability is assumed for incidental or consequential damages in connection with or arising out of information contained in this book. The Publisher shall not be liable for any special, consequential, or exemplary damages resulting, in whole or in part, from the readers' use of, or reliance upon, this material.

Independent verification should be sought for any data, advice or recommendations contained in this book. In addition, no responsibility is assumed by the publisher for any injury and/or damage to persons or property arising from any methods, products, instructions, ideas or otherwise contained in this publication.

This publication is designed to provide accurate and authoritative information with regard to the subject matter covered herein. It is sold with the clear understanding that the Publisher is not engaged in rendering legal or any other professional services. If legal or any other expert assistance is required, the services of a competent person should be sought. FROM A DECLARATION OF PARTICIPANTS JOINTLY ADOPTED BY A COMMITTEE OF THE AMERICAN BAR ASSOCIATION AND A COMMITTEE OF PUBLISHERS.

LIBRARY OF CONGRESS CATALOGING-IN-PUBLICATION DATA

Available Upon Request

ISBN: 978-1-60456-245-3

Published by Nova Science Publishers, Inc. ✛ *New York*

CONTENTS

PREFACE

In the western social structures the number permanently increases sleep more disturbedly. So already suffer more than 10% of the population from sleep awake disturbances which has to be treated urgently; 800,000 patients suffer under Sleep apnea and 25,000 under Narcolepsy (PETER 1995, PETER et al. 1995). Not diagnosed and untreatedly among others they cause on the one hand frequently subjective sorrow in the persons affected and on the other hand accident danger also increased one due to the increased daytime sleepiness or doziness in the traffic and at work (PETER et al. 1995, GERDESMEYER et al. 1997, RANDERATH et al. 1997, 1998, BUTTNER et al. 2000a and b).

Chapter 1

INTRODUCTION

The sleep medicine is a relatively young, interdisciplinary and integral orientated science. It is different from the "normal" medicine as a branch which mainly is a "day medicine" when "night medicine".

Are aware thinking and behaviour which forms a functional unit with man, experience - even the motoricity itself, be influenced by the sleep both in their quantity and in their quality. If the sleep is healthy and refreshing, himself can man meaning and intellect products into all his motor, in all its abilities and possibilities develop.

A healthy and restful sleep therefore forms the basis for the use and development of personality, the action and ability to communicate, also all psychological and medical therapeutical interventions necessary for man and therefore.

While you can compensate at the healthy sleeper sleep deficits and/or nightly impairments mostly in the following sleep period, untreated sleep disorders can lead to a chronic lack of sleep or a material change of the sleep quality.

The Sleep apnea syndrome primarily is part of these sleep disorders impairing the person affected strongly. Here is intermittent apneas which appear during the sleep. With every man some apneas can appear during the night. If they more frequently appear as five times per hour and last longer than 10 seconds, however, if perhaps changes of the brain functions and a disturbance of the sleep expiry are moreover ascertainable, then a Sleep apnea syndrome is probable.

The breath interruption phases appear in difficult cases more often than 20 times per hour. The breathing time is registered in the brain of the sleeping and overcome by a bread roll reaction (arousal). The arousal reaction is essential and protects the person affected from suffocating. By the arousal reaction, however, the sleep is disturbed itself since a transition of a deep sleep stage into an only superficial sleep takes place or which prevents deep sleep to itself. Not only the number but also the period of the breath interruption phases occurs increasingly in the further course of a disease.

From an untreated chronic apnea syndrome into heart attack and stroke as well as libido loss and impotence high blood pressure, cardiac insufficiency (reduced heart performance), arrhythmias and the amplified inclination regularly develop.

In the sleep it comes to an atony of the musculature of the nose throat room with every man. At the so-calledly obstructive Sleep apnea syndrome (OSAS) it comes the one himself to a narrow position of the throat room – as a muscle tube of more than 20 muscle couples. After the apnea a deep breath which opens the respiratory tract made narrower and gets audible as loud snoring clay comes. Sleep apnea syndrome often steps open, in large numbers (two thirds of the Apnoiker are overweight) at overweight at duration snorers at which the breath and heart reactions are hindered particularly, too.

Patients who have fallen ill with a nightly breath regulation disturbance in need of treatment, complain that they would wake up how whackedly, smashed, tiredly, during the day, are frequently tired and worn-out in the morning, would primarily fall asleep at monotonous activities like reading, television and supervision activities. Distinctive symptomatic can the fall asleep also in conversations, appear during the work or at driving a car at. The power of concentration and the memory are frequently disturbed. On the job the usual service cannot be rendered any more. Furthermore some patients describe, that they frequently suffer from headaches, have retired from social contacts increasingly already in the morning because these were too exhausting for them. Some notice a depressive atmosphere situation. A part of the patients wakes up with the feeling of the distinctive difficulty in breathing or sweating by distinctive at night at night. The partner reports about snoring extremely and nightly breath gremlins mostly. The breath gremlins of the partner often are found so dangerous that they wake the "snorer" up so that it starts to breathe again.

Chapter 2

THEORY

1. BASES OF THE SLEEP RESEARCH

1.1. What Is a Normal/Healthy Sleep?

However, what is a healthy sleep now? The phenomenon has mankind employed and fascinated simultaneously since the beginnings sleep. We can take from the traditions of the legends, fairytale, literature, philosophy and medicine that the sleep in which all body and consciousness events are put "on zero" was frequently considered a completely inactive condition. One compared the sleep with the death.

Was due to the the sleep scientifically does not examine long time since you assumed that this is a condition of reduced activity merely. The researches which started only in the middle of the 20th century reveal sleep but as an extremely active condition in which parts of the body work "on low flame" others are in turn extremely active. Many body functions are adapted subject to an approximately 24-hour rhythm, for example body temperature, hormone, gastric acid and gall production, blood pressure, heartbeat etc. to the duration of day and night. The sleep awake rhythm is also adapted to the day night rhythm with the adult person. Besides that broader shorter periodical rhythms exist with influence on the alertness degree.

In the afternoon, a second low appears concerning efficiency in which the body is prepared for quiet, for example. The midday-closing is part of everyday life in the southern countries. This silent period is sacrificed to the uninterrupted workflow most in the north and Western Europe. We can live straight away without afternoon nap, however, many people have the need at this time to have a rest.

The night sleep is divided up into five different stadia, four Non REM and a REM stage:

- One sleep stage = stage 1
- Light sleep stage = stage 2
- Middle sleep stage= stage 3
- Deep sleep stage = stage 4
- REM sleep

The sleep which finally in an approx. 5-20-minute REM phase leads starts with the one sleep stage, becomes stage 4 of stage 1 more deeply, then changes again into the light sleep after approx. 90-120 minutes. Such a sleep cycle lasts for about 90-120 minutes and will pass through about four in the course of a night until five times. Remove the amount of deep sleep with an increasing sleep duration, the REM phases increase, however.

The undisturbed expiry of this cycles is the prerequisite for a restful sleep. Differences are frequently differences persons (interindividual) ascertainably, hardly any regarding the sleep within a person (intraindividual).

Table 1. Distribution of sleep stages

Stadia	Brain current waves (EEG)	Eye muscles (EOG)	Chin muscle (EMG)	% complete sleep
Keep watch	Alpha- (8-13 Hz) and beta waves (15-35 Hz)	quick eye movement	changing muscle tension	5%
NON REM stage 1	Alpha, beta and theta waves (4-7 Hz)	slow, rolling eye movements	Muscle tension low than in the awake condition	5-10%
stage 2	sleep spindles (12-14 Hz) and K complexes	no eye movements	muscle tension low than in the awake condition	50%
stage 3/4	delta waves (1-4 Hz)	no eye movements	muscle tension low than in the awake condition	20%
REM	Beta sample with alpha and theta waves	quick eye movements	Muscle tension on zero occasional convulsions	20-25%

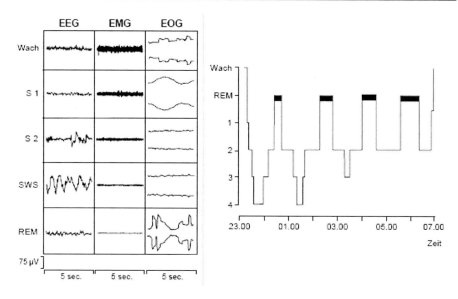

Figure 1. Sleep architecture.

Man spends about one quarter to a third of his life in the sleep. Starting out from on an average eight hours per night and a life expectancy of 80 years these are altogether 233 600 hours or approximate for 27 years.

The remaining 53 years of the life which are spent in the awake condition are influenced by the sleep quality considerably. The results of a night stayed awake through are well-known: doziness, lack of concentration and general decline in performance.

Table 2. Sleep characteristics

The sleep of a healthy young adult can be characterized as follows:
– average sleep duration per night: 6-9 hours
– number of cycles per night: 4-6
– duration of a cyklus: 90-120 minute
– share of the sleep stadia: Non REM 1 5%
Non REM 2 50%
Non REM 3 8%
Non REM 4 12%
REM 25%
– It a proportional relationship of deep sleep and REM share insists 25%.

While such a deficit can recover at the healthy sleeper in the following sleep period again, untreated sleep disorders can to a chronic lack of sleep do or a material lead changes of the sleep quality.

1.2. Sleep Disorders

The healthy sleep is disturbed, however, increasingly in today's time: The changes of the lifestyle (shift or night-work; fast food; put under stress among others) particularly in Europe, Eastern Asia and the USA (e.g. 30% of the population works at night) lead to an increase in sleeplessnesses. The increasing pressure in the professional life can result in one's not coming to the quiet any more that one in the evening or at night restlessly to and in turn what can point to other illnesses also, however, himself. So after all 40% of all depressions speak by sleeplessnesses (particularly by Insomnia) first.

Particularly in the western social structures the number permanently increases sleep more disturbedly but they are no more rareness in other cultural areas like bspw. in Eastern Europe, in the Orient or in Asia either. At present, about 60 different illnesses which appear during the sleep at night and disturb this severely are known. The *Insomnia* are part of the best known illnesses among others, the *Sleep apnea syndrome and the Narcolepsy.*

Altogether, 800,000 patients already suffer Peter 1995 in Western Europe more than 10% of the population of Sleep apnea syndromes and 25,000 to Narcolepsy from sleep awake disturbances which has to be treated urgently (PETER 1995, PETER et al. 1995).

Not diagnosed and untreatedly among others Peter et al. these illnesses cause on the one hand frequently subjective sorrow with the persons affected and on the other hand accident danger frequently also increased one due to the increased daytime sleepiness or doziness in the traffic and at work (e.g. PETER et al. 1995, GERDESMEYER et al. 1997, RANDERATH et al. 1997, 1998, BÜTTNER et al. 1999, 2000, 2001, 2002, 2003).

Outside Western Europe, North America and Australia exitieren but till now almost no sleep laboratory in which the patients concerned partly extremely can be diagnosed and treated.

1.2.1. Definition of the Sleep Disorders
Causes great difficulties to define sleep disorders exactly. In connection with this, the existence of a difference between subjective sleep need and sleep fortunes seems particularly important.

One generally defines sleep disorders "as a temporary or chronic inability to get the lot of sleep which is required for the organism to work efficiently during the day" (OBST 1989). One chronically understands a duration of at least three weeks under.

People who suffers from sleep disorders do not complain falling asleep knowledge, unpleasantly felt interruptions of the sleep expiry mainly about and about lacking relaxation. Results are frequently sleepiness, malaise, daily output weakness or/and also depression. First or particularly the results make the sleep disorders a serious problem for the persons affected. Man generally needs so much sleep, how to his well-being is required (SCHIMDT 1985, RAHM 1994).

1.2.2. Developmental History of the Classification

There are different explanation models and division criteria for the classification of sleep disorders:

- the aetiology, this one into endogenous/exogenous as well as into somatic/emotional causes
- categorized
- the appearance time
- the course
- the severity degree
- the Chronificication
- the (predominant) phenotype of the disturbance, which one in symptoms, descriptive in is subjective and registered complaints and the consequences subdivided during the day

(RAHM 1994).

Kleitmann (1939, 1963) suggested a *phenomenological subdivision* with subjective details or polygraphic methods.

- The sleep disorders were/are subdivided into three categories:
- problems in getting to sleep
- waking up early deduces
- to fall asleep with the inability again

(RAHM 1994).

Finke and Schult

+e (1970/1979) suggested a *etiological division* in the German-speaking room. sleep disorders which is characterized by exogenous or emotional reactive emergence conditions and organically conditional subdivide you into functional sleep disorders (RAHM 1994).

Karacan and Hursch (1974) as well as Parkes (1985) define *Dyssomnia* as *a generic term* which they subdivide into four categories:

- primary sleep disorders
- secondary sleep disorders
- Parasomnien and
- sleep disorders in connection with striking body functions
(RAHM 1994).

1979 published a group of American sleep researchers the Association *of* Sleep Disorders centre (ASDC) a comprehensive and detailed classification system the *"Diagnostic Classification of Sleep and Arousal Disorders"*. This found international recognition, is but for the clinical application to extensive (RAHM 1994, SCHINDLER 1994).

The American Psychiatric Association (APA) included the sleep disorders 1985 in the *DSM-III R*. It has a similar construction like the ASDC, is, however, less from subtly differentiated (HERMANN-MAURER 1990, DSM-III R 1993, RAHM 1994).

The American Sleep Disorders Association created the *ICSD ("International Classification of Sleep Disorders")* in 1990.

It contains altogether 90 different disturbance pictures. The ICSD subdivides sleep disorders into four generic terms:

- Dyssomnias, this one in intrinsische, extrinsische sleep disorders and disturbances of the circadian rhythm being distinguished
- Parasomnias
- Sleep disorderes with medically caused sleep disorders
(ICSD 1995, RAHM 1994).

The sleep disorders also were included in the manual of the *ICD-10* in 1993 (RAHM 1994, ICD-10 1995). For the development the general base got the ASDC classification borrows. The diagnostic assignment is here carried out both to psychiatric and to neurological syndromes. So the organic sleep disorders are assigned to the neurological and the non-organic one assigned to the psychiatric syndromes (PATEROK 1993, ICD-10 1995).

1.3. Summary of the Most Important Syndromes

1.3.1. Chronic Primary Insomnia

The *chronic primary Insomnia* arises from the interaction of emotional physiological "Hyperarousal" with a "learnt misconduct". It is suspected that the sleeplessness by a disturbed excitement balance ("Arousal") is triggered due to a cognitive, physiological or emotional excitement refreshment. Switching off knowledge and behaviours sleep disturbing konditionierte do not determine the cognitive factors. One about or are a sub-excitement of autonomous functions at a physiological level responsibly. Disturbing emotional factors arise either from certain personal characteristics (timidity, strain) or from reactively conditional situations (stress, conflicts).

Most prevalence examinations define *Insomnia* merely as a sleeplessness. Under this criterion the frequency is in the western industrial countries between 20-30 % in which about 10-15 % have fallen ill with heavy and thus treatment worthy sleeplessnesses.

Every fourth one already suffers in Western Germany from *Insomnia* (one or by sleeplessnesses) which is not triggered by outer causes. About 15% of the population feel tiredly and through this impaired in their efficiency often or always during the day.

Due to the high illness instalments the *Insomnia* frequently is not taken seriously by the persons affected and the attending doctors as illness. Only approx. 15-20 % the fallen ill ask for professional help although approximately a fifth of all patients of a general medical practice has fallen ill with a sleeplessness. Suffering a third in neurological clinical complexes and in psychiatric approx. three quarters of the patients under a disturbed sleep (Berger et al. 1993, HAJAK and RÜTHER 1995).

The therapy of the *Insomnia* is based on a multimodal therapy concept since several causes independent of each other can always play a part in the emergence of *an Insomnia*. Every single cause can HAJAK et al. require a special treatment (HAJAK et al. 1992, HAJAK and RÜTHER 1995).

Not pharmacological therapy approaches cover mainly behaviour therapeutical approaches, expansion procedures and psychological treatment besides the base methods of the clearing up and advice on the basis of different therapy forms.

1.3.2. Sleep Apnea Syndrome

Sleep apnea syndromes are complex syndromes whose causes are multifaktoriell. Primarily anatomical and central nervous changes as well as adiposity are part of the causes. *Sleep apnea syndrome*s are indicated by nightly breath gremlins. Pathophysiological it comes inpiratorical for an approach of the pharyngealen walls until the collapse (LEVY et al. 1994). A reduction or adjusting the breath current for the time being although furthermore thorakale and abdominelle breath movements are executed result from it.

Table 3. Characteristics of the chronic primary Insomnia

On this basis can be divided up into two categories simplifying the symptomatic:	
Sleep complaints	Day state

1. night sleep:
   – too superficial
   – easy
   – short
   – restless
   – not restful
 	
 2. long awake times:
   – before falling asleep
   – after a awakening at night
 	
 3. numerous short on-awake phases.
 	
 4. subjective sleep impairments
 	
 Also subjective sleep impairments are often connected with the clinical symptomatic.
 	
 The subjective sleep expiry is partly undisturbed, however, gets nevertheless as described little or not restfully.
 	
 Sometimes provable changes in the fine structure of the sleep are found in the polysomnography; no objective results often exist, however.
	1. day state partly not impaired:
	   – frequent but under a strong exhaustion and
	   – day sleepiness
	   – Concentration and efficiency reduced
	   – general malaise and drive weakness
	
	 2. in addition frequent:
	   – muscle pains
	   – irritability
	   – depressive ill-feelings
	   – anxiety
	
	 There is frequently a discrepancy between the vigilance measured objectively and the subjective assessment of the insomnics.
	
	 Tiredness tests often yielded a bad sleep readiness on the day although the persons affected suffered from subjective sleepiness. Even the healthy ones partly surpass it with its alertness (increased share of fast frequencies in the alpha ribbon).
	
	 The increased physiological excitement standard before particularly and at the beginning of the sleep period promotes or solves at many Insomniapatienten the inability to sleep.

With SAS patients the opening is therefore made narrower to the windpipe at the tongue approach so that at the breathing the air cannot stream unhinderedly into the lungs. In the sleep the opening completely shuts itself off. For 10 to 60 seconds, partial still longer, the breathing then stops. The body reacts with a short, unconscious bread roll reaction. This can happen 50-60 times in the hour. So it comes that the person affected is cheated snoring out ouf the restful deep sleep and dream sleep phases.

Particularly the threatening subsequent illnesses spitefully are up to the heart attack or stroke, caused by the permanent oxygen insufficient supply of the brain.

So 80% of all 30-60-year-old patients suffer from all sorts of results with SAS among others at excessive daytime sleepiness and a duration attention reduced, in addition. Resulting from it it comes to performance losses both professional and in the ability to stock motor vehicles. Accidents or almost accidents are therefore frequently result of this reduced efficiency by falling asleep at the steering wheel. Nightly arousals are triggering sleep fragmentation as well as hypoxies for this with consecutive.

Table 4. Characteristics of the Sleep apnea syndrome

Nightly symptomatics	Daytime symptomatics
– apneas – snoring strongly – hypoxies (anoxies) – sleep fragmentation – reduction of the slow sleep wave stadia 3 and 4+REM sleep – nightly hypertonia – nightly heart conditions+heart attack	– sweating and muzziness after waking up/get up – extensive daytime sleepiness+second sleep – loss of intellectual abilities – (e.g. deficits in vigilance; cognitive functions) – hypertonia during the day (later than the nightly one) – heart conditions+heart attack during the day (~) – apoplex – loss of the libido+disturbance of the erection – pains of head; neck; shoulder and back – depressive symptoms

Endangered but also other street road users are but not only the fallen ill. So about 15 to 20 per cent of all accidents decline to a simple oversleepiness according to the statistics in the goods traffic (the numbers for the passenger transport are unknown due to the data protection definitions, however, also will turn out very high presumably if one takes into account subjective self-assessments of patients). The second sleep is more frequently still than alcohol the most frequent cause of an accident with that.

These accidents cause therefore on the one hand considerable sorrow or frequent also suffering with the involvierten persons or on the other hand however also considerable financial losses (damages to property, economic damage).

The prevalence of the *Sleep apnea syndrome (SAS)* cannot be obviously found out due to the different norm and limiting values. It is nevertheless possible to make quite reliable statements on the frequency of these illnesses. Von SAS is mainly the male sex concernedly. A relationship of 95 : 5 (stands up), to the menopause men: women, till now, a possible connection with the testosterone mirror is not cleared yet. 1-5 % of the population have presumably fallen ill with OSAS in the western world. 25-30 % Sleep apnea syndromes were described at patients with hypertonia and 35-45 % with patients with on the left heart-failure. The SAS frequency increases with an advancing age and reaches their peak at the age from 50 to 70 years.

The *Sleep apnea syndrome* itself can by means of a device connected to a nose mask, the *nasal Continuous positives Airway pressing aurochs,* short, this according to the excess pressure principle works, be treated nCPAP. The nCPAP device blows room air into the nose, the pressure prevents the seal of the windpipe and with that the breath gremlins and the oxygen waste resulting from it. At first it comes to a normalization of the sleep profile, i.e. to an increase of the essential deep sleep shares as well as to a sleep phase normalization after that. In the further course it then comes himself to an improvement in the daytime symptomatic, i.e. attention, concentration, mental and increase physical capacity again, too. Also the accompanying and subsequent illnesses (e.g of cardiovascular, neurological or psychiatric illnesses) improve or stabilize themselves late, i.e. after approx. a ½ year.

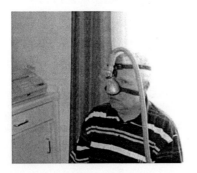 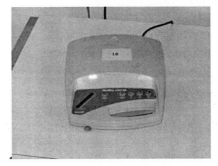

Figure 2. nCPAP equipment and its use.

The causes or the triggering factors of the *Sleep apnea syndrome* are unsolved to this day, what aggravates its treatment. So the method of treatment (nCPAP) described above is very simple and nevertheless only a method which requires a lifelong treatment effectively does not make a cure possible, however. Aggravating the compliance of the patients is additionally, due to the machine-aided method (be self-supporting) the himself the mask connected to the nCPAP device (particularly younger men) considerably partly feel restricted in its quality of life there.

1.3.3. Narcolepsy

Narcolepsy is a causally still unknown malfunction of the sleep/awake-regulating centres in the brain with an invincible one sleep inclination by sleep amounts suddenly appearing which reveals itself. These attacks are a distinctive, if also not absolutely mandatory feature of the suffering. The disturbance of the "sleep and awake structure" also shows itself in additional malfunctions.

The illness was described by the French neurologist and psychiatrists Gélineau for the first time to 1880.

In the classic neurology and psychiatry books does not become *the Narcolepsy* at all or mentions only very only just although it is not at all so rare. The exact prevalence only can be valued in the general population since there are no methodically faultless studies. Great differences exist in its appearance frequency.

So a frequency of 0.16 % becomes indicated one of 0.0002 % for Japan and unlike this for Israel. Central Europe (0.006 %) and the USA (0.06-0.1 %) are located in the middle. The details on the sex distribution do not agree among the different authors. So a part indicates a larger illness frequency with men (LEU 1992) while other authors report about a sex uniform distribution (HOHAGEN and SCHÖNBRUNN 1992).

The first clinical symptoms of *the Narcolepsy* usually manifest themselves during the puberty or shortly after this. The illness peak is frequently located in the middle of the third decade of life. However, it first manifestations appear, also in front of 10th year of life or after the 50th year of life (HOHAGEN and SCHÖNBRUNN 1992, LEU 1992, MAYER et al. 1993). Most examinations showed that approx. 2/3 of the patients suffered from sleep paralyses to Kataplexien, approx. 1/3 of hypnagogen hallucinations and approx. 1/4. There was the "narcoleptic tetrade" approximately 10% of the cases. The frame is minted completely at approx. 15% the fallen ill (HOHAGEN and SCHÖNBRUNN 1992, Praxis-Information 04/1992).

Table 5. Characteristics of the Narcolepsy

The combination of the four main symptoms is called "narkoleptic tetrade" (GLASZ 1996).
o   excessive daytime sleepincss/a one sleep inclination/imperative one sleep attacks o   cataplexias o   hypnagoge hallucination o   sleep paralysis
Broader symptoms:
o   shortening of the REM latency until Sleep*Onset* REM sleep periods o   arrangement for low blood pressure and a tendentious flattening out of the body temperature curve
The frame of the Narcolepsy is determined by six cardinal symptoms:

o   imperative one sleep attacks and day sleepiness increased
o   cataplexias (affective loss of tonus)
o   hypnagoge hallucinations
o   sleep paralysis (dissoziiertes wake up)
o   disturbed night sleep
     o   waking up frequently
     o   Sleep*Onset*REM and
     o   increased changes of sleep stages
     o   automatic actions/behaviour

The causes of the *Narcolepsy* are largely unknown to this day although this illness was described over 100 years ago for the first time (MEIER-EWERT 1989, LEU 1992, GEISLER 1993, BORCK 1995, GLASZ 1996).

You prove, that genes play a large role in the illness. Numerous studies illustrate a family accumulation in which this also shows considerable fluctuations between the different nationalities (GEISLER 1993, BORCK 1995, GLASZ 1996). Furthermore a strong connection between the HLA antigen DR2 and *Narcolepsy* was discovered. It has this gene combination only approx. 25% of the healthy European population, unlike this exists to 98-100 % at Narcolepsypatienten (LEU 1992, GEISLER 1993, ZIMMER 1993, BORCK 1995, GLASZ 1996).

Since *Narcolepsy* is not "curable" to itself, the treatment restricts itself to the elimination or at least alleviation of its consequences. By a sensible customization of the way of life and at the same time a treatment carefully coordinated individually with medicine the quality of life improved quite considerably and the professional ability can be got.

Some Narcolepsy ailing ones get relief from so-called "alternative cures", such as acupuncture, acupressure etc., at least with the advantage of lower or missing side effects.

2. MEANING AND FUNCTION OF THE SLEEP LABORATORIES

With the represented above particularly with the three syndromes introduced exemplarily chosen by me gets, that illnesses to be taken seriously sleeping sicknesses represent, clear which has to be treated absolutely and that sleep laboratories are indispensable and necessary in today's societies.

Sleep laboratories therefore serve as a matter of priority the diagnostics, therapy and therapy control of sleep diseases different nightly (e.g. of the diagnosis epilepsy appearing only at night). To be able to diagnose, to treat and to investigate the existing sleeplessnesses or sleep diseases, a nightly examination, polysomnography, is indispensable.

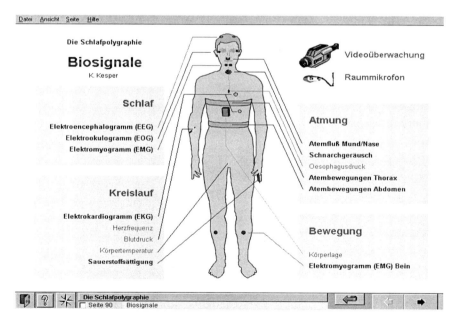

Figure 3. Polysomnography.

Being the heart tones, brain currents and leg convulsions, the breathing volume and the oxygen content in the blood as well as the snoring noises recorded by means of electrodes at this.

Besides the nightly polysomnography frequently further examinations are nessary for the diagnostics and/or therapy course control, belong to them particularly with professional drivers. Among others:

o   Sleepiness scales
o   Measurement of sleepiness
o   Measurement of vigilance.

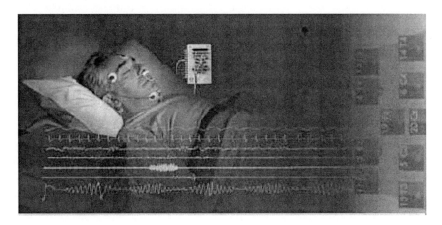

Figure 4. Nightly wiring in the sleep laboratory.

Further main focuses of the work of the sleep laboratories are the investigation *of the accompanying and subsequent illnesses* of the sleep-related illnesses particularly on attention, concentration deficits, losses, the mental one and physical capacity, sexual disturbances, cardiovascular, neurological or psychiatric illnesses at SAS, Narcolepsy and/or Restleg syndrome and its treatment possibilities.

Frequently biol physiological fundamental research and the examination of the so-called daytime symptomatics of the illnesses mentioned above are stand in the centre concerning the excessive daytime sleepiness, the reduced duration attention and the cognitive efficiency reduced. These aspects get explosive by the consequences resulting from them frequently, mentioned above already, the increased accident danger, accidents or almost accidents by falling asleep at the steering wheel in the traffic and/or at work.

Arises also inevitably that research a multidisciplinary attempt at reason lies the sleep medical? Important is particularly the cooperation with the traffic medical one and neuropsychological research and development but also with facilities or ministries concerning traffic engineering.

Chapter 3

THE OBSTRUCTIVE SLEEP APNEA SYNDROME

1. HISTORICAL SUMMARY

Sleep to untimeliness as a phenomenon which puts a challenge to the clinician thinking interdisciplinarily today was already in the ancient times known. Already in the antiquity became the duration doziness of that obese Dionysus, tyrant of Herakleia, which became a slave on every occasion to the sleep and could be woken only with pinpricks again described (KRYGER 1983). The 1836 of Charles Dickens which permanently fell asleep on his coach box, Burwell describes the syndrome described by it for the first time in 1956 the "Posthumous paper of the Pickwick club" "described Fat Joe" with the symptoms adiposity by magna, hypersomnolence and alveolar hypoventilation with cor pulmonale as Pickwick syndrome (BURWELL et al. 1956) in the dependence to into. Jung and Kuhlo recognized apneas about 10 years later than a moment important to pathogenetic in the development of this syndrome which are intermittent and appearing in the sleep only. Furthermore you described the drastic recovery by the tracheostomy (YOUNG and KUHLO 1965).

Scientific examinations within the following 20 years led to a quick increase in knowledge concerning epidemiological meaning, pathophysiology, diagnostics, differential diagnostics and therapy possibilities of the Sleep-related breathing disturbances.

Basic work came from GUILLEMINAULT et al. at this time. He stamped for the first time the concept Sleep apnea syndrome in 1976 which contains complexe diseases, which underlies causal the Sleep apnea.

First surprising epidemiological data brought about the examinations of LAVIE (1983) and LUGARESI (1983) as well as the country study of PETER

(1986) which had for the first time been carried out by means of the itinerantly usable portable cassette recorder systems.

Against the background of the therapeutical possibilities assessed at first completely unsatisfactorily at Sleep apnea the report introduced by SULLIVAN (1981) on the effectiveness of the nightly therapy meant with nCPAP (nasal Continuous positives Airway pressing aurochs) at an obstructive apnea unite important progress. Following experiences with the domestically applicable nCPAP therapy in the different sleep centres established this therapy form to the most important one quickly and furthermore produced impulses for the far-reaching clarification this one for OSA of substantial pathogenetic mechanisms.

2. DEFINITION

Sleep apnea syndromes are complex syndromes whose causes are multifaktoriell. You are indicated by nightly breath gremlins (cf. Table 6). Pathophysiological it comes inspiratorical for an approach of the pharyngealen walls until the collapse (LEVY et al. 1994). A reduction or a adjusting the breath current for the time being although furthermore thorakale and abdominale breath movements are executed result from it.

Table 6. Indices of the Sleep apnea syndrome (Meier-Ewert, 1989)

Index	Explanation
Desaturation index	The Desaturation index says the O2 repletion curve of the hemoglobins how frequently sinks in an hour by at least 4%.
Apnea index	The Apnea index indicates the number of the apnea phases/hours.
Breathing disturbance index	The Breathing disturbance index indicates the number of apnea and hypopnea phases/hours.

There are numerous definitions of which two are outstanding:

- *the Stanford definition* (called also classic definition) and

A Sleep apnea syndrome is diagnosed if during a 7-hour polygraphic night derivation, with a duration of more, at least 30 apnoephasen appear into REM and NREM sleep as 10 s of which some regularly recur in the NREM sleep.

- *the Marburg definition*

A Sleep apnea syndrome is diagnosed if in a 7-hour polygraphic night derivation more than 10 apnea phases/hours appear outside the REM sleep of more as 10 s with a duration.
(MEIER-EWERT 1989, FAUST, M. et al. 1992).

3. DIAGNOSTIC CRITERIA AND CLINICAL PHENOTYPE

3.1. Diagnostic Criteria

The Sleep apnea syndrome is a complaint picture which as a rule is caused by apneas during the sleep and is primarily indicated by a distinctive daytime sleepiness up to the one sleep compulsion (second sleep). Besides that there still are a number of broader symptoms and subsequent illnesses.

On-bread roll reactions, so-called arousals (as an automatic alarm reaction of the body) which usually is not perceived by the persons affected, however, consciously, repeated lead the apneas to an oxygen insufficient supply and to. Result of the on-bread roll reactions is a not restful sleep, in turn what leads to the typical distinctive daytime sleepiness. The Sleep apnea syndrome belongs to the Dyssomnias, i.e. the medically meaningful sleep disorder.

3.2. Symptomatic

A Sleep apnea is speaking if in the sleep an apnea appears with a minimum duration of 10 s. Under the concept apnea become both the pure apnea, (i.e. the suspension of the breath current to mouth and nose) and also the hypopnea, (i.e. a hypoventilation with waste of the oxygen repletion of the arterial blood by at least 4% compared with the initial value) subsumes. As Apnea index the number of the apneas per hours sleep time is defined. At an Apnea index of 10 must be started out from a clinically relevant Sleep apnea (KONIETZKO et al. 1993a).

The sleep of the OSAS patient is characterized by waking up in large numbers and Arousals. The deep sleep phases 3, 4 and the REM sleep are reduced, the sleep phases 1 through and 2 increases, however (MEIER-EWERT 1989, FAUST et al. 1992, LUND 1994).

The sleep is not at all therefore restful and the OSAS patients feel in the next morning unausgeruht and fall through. These sleep anomalities lead to sleepiness and sleep attacks during the day. The patients after awakening morningly are often confused, sweaty or they partly complain over headaches as well as over neck, shoulder, cross and backache about depressive symptoms and losses of intellectual abilities. In the outside case history reports partners mostly about loudly snoring, breath gremlins as well as increased daytime sleepiness (MEIER-EWERT 1989, LUND 1994, ROHMFELD et al. 1994; Table 7).

Table 7. Symptoms of the Sleep apnea syndrome

Conducting symptoms	Frequent symptoms	Optional symptoms
o Snoring o Daytime sleepiness/-doziness with increased one sleep inclination o nightly breathing times o Sleeplessnesses (by Arousal sleep fragmentation)	o restless sleep o morning headaches o Lack of concentration o cognitive deficits o lacking efficiency o Irritability o Personality changes o Inclination to depressive ill-feeling	o Night sweat o Increase in weight o Libido loss/impotence o Alcohol intolerance

This increased daytime sleepiness and a one sleep inclination partly lead to considerable fluctuatations of vigilance and possible also to cognitive losses. With event correlated potentials (ECP) the cognitive functions can be checked and judged with neurophysiologischen methods (DUSCHA et al. 1995, MARSUPIAL and HAAN 1995).

By definition the periodical apnea phases last for at least 10 seconds. The apneas get clinically relevant if at least five Apnoezyklen per hour appear. The oxygen content also sinks strongly in the blood at this time. It comes to on the right heart loads and pulmonaler hypertonia as results. Furthermore libido loss or impotence often appears (RÜHLE 1993, Lund 1994).

In addition, the OSAS also arouses a whole number of cardiorespiratoric consequences:

- disturbances of the intrapulmonalen gas interchange with a rezidivided oxygen partial pressure drop and a carbon dioxide partial rise in pressure
- malicious dynamic consequences (e.g. arterial and/or pulmonalarterial hypertonia and cardiac insufficiency)
- cardiac activity tannin wrestled
- increase of the oxygen consumption of the myocard (dangerous in patients with coronary heart disease)

- nightly arrhythmias (sinusatriale and atrioventriculare blockings)
- polyglobulias
- increased risk for myocard infarkts and apoplex

(BECKER et al. 1993, LANGANKE et al. 1993, LUND 1994).

Furthermore OSAS persons affected are also High risk patients at operations (PENTZ 1993).

3.3. Clinical Phenotype

There is a whole number of transition forms between snoring physically harmless regularly and the heavy OSAS. However, this does not mean that every snorer as heavy Sleep apnea patients ends. The OSAS is marked with breathing times by a snoring very irregularly. These two symptoms are usually watched by the partner. The breathing times lead to bread roll reactions ("arousals"). You can be very frequent and disrupt sleep architecture lastingly, what polysomnographic represents a main feature for the diagnostics. The patient then suffers from a daytime sleepiness with a one sleep inclination in all possible situations. The younger the patient is, the more soonly he can compensate for disturbed sleep architecture, however. This also only can speak into concentration disturbances as in the case of children. A long time damage is always put, however.

The appearance of periodical apneas is the reason that the restful sleep of the OSAS patient is disturbed (primarily reduction of the delta and REM sleep share, sleep fragmentation). The sleep phases 1 and 2 increase, these phases 3 and 4 are reduced (MEIER-EWERT 1989).

Since the sleep is not at all restful, a very strong one sleep inclination which is coupled with a removal of the efficiency follows during the day. Partly the Sleep apnea patients after awakening morningly are often forgotten or complain, confused, over headaches as well as over neck, shoulder, cross and backache. In the literature personality changes, impotence, nightly enuresis, become outbursts of rage besides these complaints or symptoms and mentions depression or feelings of anxiety (MATHIS 1988). A professional and social decline of the patient has to be watched often. The partner reports most about snoring loudly, breath gremlins as well as daytime sleepiness increased (MEIER-EWERT 1989).

The existence of a daytime symptomatic is a necessary criterion for the diagnosis of a Sleep apnea syndrome.

Declines in performance at Sleep apnea patients can prove in neuropsychological methods particularly in the area of the attention the let oneself be seen the attention, the concentration fortunes, the vigilance, the memory (proved verbally more considerably than figured), which serves the check of the frontal brain function in tasks and in the affective area (FINDLEY et al. 1999, 2000, GEORGE et al. 1999, 2000, WEESS et al. 1998, BÜTTNER et al. 2000a, 2000b).

At his study REDLINE (1997) noticed that Sleep apnea patients show impairments backwards with a mild OSA syndrome (AHI 10-20) in visual vigilance tasks, in the working memory and in the Number Repeating Test (back out), however no differences opposite a control group regarding information processing speed, ascertainable test is, Trail Making Test and Wisconsin Card Sorting Test.

FEUERSTEIN (1997) found increased difficulties of events automated when initiating new cognitive processes and simultaneous problems in holding back as well as takes a tendency toward perseveration by OSAS patients together under thinking operations which are steered by the frontal rag primarily. Also in this study deficits of studying of verbal and visual let themselves be seen.

VALENCIA-FLORES (1996) built the hypothesis that the reduced vigilance is responsible only for a part of the symptoms watched at the OSA syndrome (primarily for a reduced verbal studying fortune) while the effects of the chronic nightly hypoxy (reduced oxygen) are responsible for impairments in the area of the attention. This explained to Valencia-Flores that the verbal studying fortune improves primarily by an effective therapy at short notice.

VERSTRAETEN (1996) did not find any performance differences at the comparison of the neuropsychological efficiency of OSAS patients with the one of patients who suffer from a primary Insomnia. It therefore becomes the available cognitive difficulties from it primarily on the unsatisfactory quality and insufficient quantity of the sleep led back, primarily the lack of Delta and REM sleep many other studies which proves the opposite, however, exist.

4. FORMS OF THE SLEEP APNEA SYNDROMES

The Sleep apnea syndromes (cf. Figure 5) become the apnea phases subdivided into this with the localisation:

- obstructive Sleep apnea syndrome
- central Sleep apnea syndrome
- mixed Sleep apnea syndrome.

An inspiratorical obstruction of this one lies in *the obstructive* Sleep apnea syndrome epiglottical oropharynx and epipharynx, at this sistiert the breath gas river at continual breath excursions of abdomens (belly) and thorax (chest) due to the collapsing of the upper air routes. Thorax and abdomen movements typically appear contrarily (paradoxically).

The consequence is a desaturation in turn what leads for an activation of the breath musculature and about the activation of mechanoreceptorsof also the throat musculature (OKABE et al. 1994). About the hypoxy (LEUENBERGER et al.) futhermore the sympatical nervous system (SHIMIZU et al. 1997) and the medullar respiratory centre are activated.

By this broad activation it comes to a arousal which is indicates by the change in an easier sleep stage (EEG) as well as a short-term motor activation. The apnea is ended through this, a short-term compensatorical hyperventilation follows. At a serious Sleep apnea a normalization of the oxegen repetion frequently is not reached, however, since the time period is too short simply up to the appearance of the next apnea.

These leading the apnea phases limiting arousals in their accumulation OSAS patients to a sleep fragmentation and therefore for a change of the sleep profile with reduction of the depression and REM sleep share with one more or decrease distinctive loss of the relaxation function of the sleep.

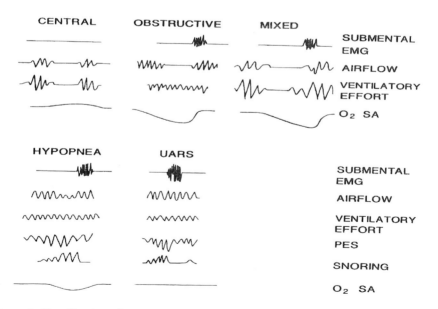

Figure 5. Classification of apneas.

The central Sleep apnea syndrome arises from apneas at an open respiratory tract. All breath movements are missing, the breath current is adjusted for the time being.

At the *mixed* Sleep apnea syndrome an obstructive one follows the part of the central apnea. The amplitudes of the thorax and abdomen excursions are in the obstructive part increases.

The obstructive Sleep apnea syndrome most frequently appears (MEIER-EWERT 1989).

5. EPIDEMIOLOGY AND COURSE

Sleep apnea syndromes are an illness happening frequent. Approx. 1-5 % is of the population affected by them (OSLON et al. 1995, PHILLIPSON and REMMERS 1989); however, men are age dependent much frequent than women (approx. ten times frequent; FISCHER et al. 1994). The most important predispositions for the development of the Sleep apnea syndrome represent the age (> 40 years) and the adiposity (BMI > 28) besides the sex (KISELAK et al. 1993, LEVINSON et al. 1993, OLSON et al. 1995, RAUSCHER et al.).

a) Prevalence

The prevalence of the obstructive Sleep apnea syndrome (OSAS) cannot be obviously found out due to the different norm and limiting values (FAUST et al. 1992). It is nevertheless possible to make quite reliable statements on the frequency of these illnesses. The male sex is mainly affected by the apnea syndromes. A relationship of approximately 95 : 5 (stands up), to the menopause men : women, till now, a possible connection with the testosterone mirror is not cleared yet.

Sleep apnea syndrome has fallen ill with Sleep apnea in the western world presumably 1-5 % of the population, according to the American Sleep Disorders Association exists at least 1% and manifested at most 2%. 25-30 % of obstructive Sleep apnea syndrome were described at patients with hypertonia and 35-45 % with patients with on the left heart-failure. The frequency of Sleep apnea syndrome increases with an advancing age and reaches its peak at the age from 50 to 70 years (MEIER-EWERT 1989, ENGFER and MEIER-EWERT 1990, FAUST et al. 1992, BAUER et al. 1995, KLUTMANN et al. 1995).

b) Predisposing Factors

In the literature five predisposing factors are found mainly for the obstructive Sleep apnea syndrome:

- a respiratory tract narrow part due to an anatomical anomality of the nasopharyngeal area
- the influence of alcohol, sedativa and painkillers (of beta blockers unsolved)
- one infection of the upper respiratory tract or a chronic, allergic rhinitis
- strong overweight
- thyroid gland diseases, acromegaly as well as neurological illnesses with bulbar amounts which have a narrowing of the upper respiratory tract the consequence

(DAMM et al. 1995, LUND 1996).

The overweight is a meaningful risk factor for the obstructive Sleep apnea syndrome (OSAS). More than 60% of the OSAS patients are strongly adipose. However, or normal weight does not exclude an OSAS (MEIER-EWERT 1989, KONIETZKO et al. 1993a).

c) Factors Illness Triggering

The obstructive Sleep apnea syndrome is triggered by *pathophysiological* factors. Particularly four factors can cause a limitation or a collapse. Each of these factors,

- the pharyngeal below pressure and the pharyngeal collapsing
- the limitation or transfer of the lumen
- the skelettalen changes
- the activity or the tonus of the upper respiratory tract
- the functional and structural factors are alone for a pharyngealen collapse insufficient, in a combination but can trigger obstructions

(HOCHBAN 1995, DUCHNA et al. 1995).

* Pharyngeal below pressure and pharyngeal collapsing

The airflow and the resistance of the nose opening or another functional narrow place determine the intrapharyngealen pressure during the inspiration. Into dependence of these two factors a below pressure arises (in accordance with Bernoullically law) opposite the surroundings, this has an effect on all collapsing pharynx parts.

The below pressure extent which leads to the complete collapse is unknown till now. Elasticity and collapsing influence the consequences of the below atmospheric pressure. As an alternative to it you discuss also about a higher respiratory tract resistance above the glottis. But not only the respiratory tract resistance and the elasticity of the pharynx arouse the collapse inclination of the pharynx, the weight also has a decisive share.

The symptoms of the sleep apnea are reduced primarily by a reduction of the pharyngeal collapsing (HOCHBAN 1995).

* Limitation of the lumen

Pathological changes often lead to the limitation or transfer of the lumen. The elastic pharyngeale lumen is subject to predominantly dynamic processes at opening and seal. These can be compensated for in sitting up with an additional mechanical transfer. In the sleep, however, an additional mechanical transfer leads to the seal to a decompensation and through this. Even situation changes do not have only influence on the respiratory tract resistance but also on the lumen. The pharyngeale lumen is the smallest in the supine position, in the side position it enlarges significantly and it is the biggest in sitting. Situation changes let a snorer seldom become an OSAS patients but these can the other way round reduce the apneas (HOCHBAN 1995).

* Skeleton ale changes

An anatomical base for pharyngeal obstructions is the skeleton of the face skull at which the soft parts of the pharynx are fixated. The tongues and musculature of mouth ground must actively be contracted more at skelettaler reserves of the lower jaw (dolichofacial face type [cf. Figure 6]) and mandibular retrognaty to keep the pharyngeale lumen open. This is particularly if the jaw angle is very big or flat valid so that dolichofacial face type (receding chin due to reserves of the lower jaw) arises, a vertical.

In this situation a rotation leads in the jaw joint for an additional dorsal shift. Due to this skelettalen position of the lower jaw it comes to a narrowing of the pharyngeal lumen and also more easily to a mouth opening e.g. if the chewing musculature tires during the sleep (HOCHBAN 1995).

The skelettal changes of the face frequently arise when it comes during the growth to a transferred nose breathing. These dentofacial changes often arise (= adenoidal facies) by adenoidal growth which represents the most frequent reason for the hindered nose breathing. Persisting transfer of the upper respiratory tract then supplies this of early childhood

- a consecutive chronic mouth breathing
- an unphysiologischen face muscle use as well as
- functional influences on it face jaw development
(HOCHBAN 1995).

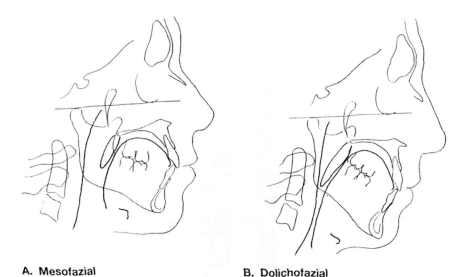

A. Mesofazial   **B. Dolichofazial**

Figure 6. Face typs – Cephalometry.

Activity or Tonus of the upper respiratory tract musculature

All anatomical defects and inaccessibilities which lead to a pharyngeal collaps due to the inspiratorischen below atmospheric pressure are usually compensated for by specific activation of pharyngeal musculature of the ZNS (provided that no central nervous disturbances exist). These compensating compensations concern the intrinsische pharynx, the tongue-bone, the palates as well as the complete chewing musculature. The musculature of the upper respiratory tract activated over reflex trains also causes the active opening of the pharynx apart from keeping open if it is kollabiert. Not only anatomical factors

but particularly also the muscle activity intending the respiratory tract resistance
and leading to differences between OSA patients and healthy. Oscillatory pressure
fluctuations lead to a stimulation of the respiratory tract musculature and with that
a keeping the air routes open in the Pharynx. The obstructive Sleep apnea partly
arises from the loss of these reflexes (HOCHBAN 1995).

d) Progression and Stages of Development

An increased daytime sleepiness is the characteristic symptom of the Sleep
apnea syndrome. The fallen ill she knows herself that, during the day, they
frequently fall asleep, disturbs this less than her surroundings, though. A doctor
visit is usually carried out only on operating the partner or the supervisor. About
60% of the Sleep apnea patients have overweight.

On questioning reporting the patients about snoring strongly and a awakening
with suffocation feeling and tachycardias. Nightly suffocation amounts which is
ended by a snoring explosively indicate the partners (inside), in addition. A fall
asleep quick evening, a restless and little restful sleep, morning start-up problems
and headaches frequently appear furthermore.

In the early stages of development the internal examination turns out normal
mostly.

Finding himself internally frequent at an advanced illness

- overweight (adiposity)
- arterial hypertonia
- cardiactases
- chronification of sleep dependent arrhythmias (e.g. Asystoles, Sine
  arrhythmia, Bradycardia and Tachycardia)
- pulmonal hypertonia
- diabetes mellitus
- arteriosclerosis
- polyglobulie.

One often does not find any on-due dates at the clinical neurological
examination (apart from adiposity) since the increased daytime sleepiness is not
always minted strongly (MEIER-EWERT 1989, BRAUS et al. 1995,
DERTINGER et al. 1995, HÖRSTENSMEYER et al. 1995, GLOSSNER-
KLEISER et al. 1995b).

In the advanced stage OSAS conditional heart attacks and/or strokes also frequently appear.

The patients partly snore already since their childhood. There also can be the overweight since the childhood or the adolescence. As a rule, year of life appears, however, a sudden increase in weight between the 30th and the 50th can use an increased daytime sleepiness to this but also with a delay from years or decades simultaneously (MEIER-EWERT 1989).

6. AETIOLOGY AND PATHOGENESIS

6.1. Aetiology

Primarily genetic, central nervous and hormonal changes are part of the causes but as well as adiposity also anatomical.

The OSAS appears family in large numbers. As additional risk factors male sex, menopause, overweight and alcohol and medicine consumption increased are described. Reason for the breathing times is a temporary complete seal of the upper air routes in the pharynx by an anatomical instability probably provided genetically. An increased kompensatorische needs neuromuscular activity this instability which is discontinued in the sleep and possibly causes the corresponding pharyngeal collaps.

6.2. Pathogenesis

Cause of OSAS is the seal of the upper respiratory tract which leads to a breathing time. This is followed by a bread roll reaction. The severity degree of the OSAS is dependent on the number and duration of breathing times. Younger patients have shorter breathing times closed seen statistically, from time to time such, which hardly leads to a waste of the oxygen repletion while in patients the breathing times get longer and lead to heavier oxygen desaturation with a course of a disease lasting long. The breathing time is reason for the bread roll reaction and for the desaturation. The bread roll reactions which lead to a disturbed sleep architecture are therefore primarily responsible for the complaints of the patients. The desaturations are secondary and can at Sleep apnea syndrome existing for a long time particularly if the oxygen repletion which vigilance and the intellectual efficiency impair is deep also on the day. The not restful sleep leads to the

physical disturbance. The oxygen desaturations then frequently lead secondarily
to cardiovascular problems (cf. Figure 7).

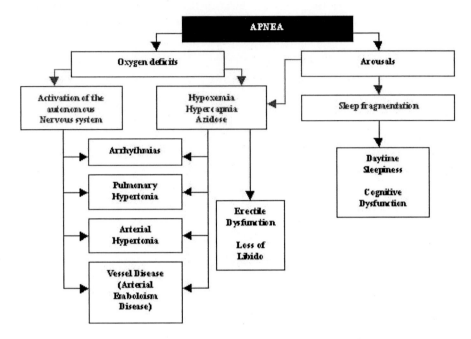

Figure 7. Way of working of the Apneas.

Sleep apnea syndromes arise from oropharyngeal obstructions, alveolar
hypoventilations and sleep fragmentation are regarded as a "pathogenetic Triassic
Period" of the Sleep apnea syndromes, particularly the obstructive one and the
mixed one (KONIETZKO et al. 1993a).

a) Oropharyngeal Obstructions

The obstruction of the oropharynx frequently leads to alveolar
hypoventilations particularly when the activity of the breath musculature is
continued. A changed blow volume in addition, it comes to great intrathoracal
pressure fluctuations, these in turn have an effect on the return current of the
venous blood and cause a changing filling of the heart and by which. These
changes can do to hypertonia at a combination with the hypoventilation-related
hypoxamias in the small and/or great circulation, lead to arrhythmias and heart
insuffizienz (KONIETZKO et al. 1993a).

b) Alveolar Hypoventilations

Apneas cause alveolar hypoventilationen whose extent strongly depends on the number and the duration of breath gremlins. Precapillar pulmonale hypertonia as well as hypoxamia and hyperkapnia in the arterial blood are the results of these hyperventilations (KONIETZKO et al. 1993a, ALTMEIER et al. 1995).

c) Sleep Fragmentation

A mechanism going off central more nervously, by reflex action ends the apneas. In the course of an apnea phases the hyperkapnie and the hypoxia stimuli permanently increase until they finally trigger an arousal (a bread roll stimulus). A flatter sleep stage gets recognizable in the EEG.

The arousal causes a permanent change of the vigilance, this one, re-rum causes a sleep fragmentation. A serious physiological sleep structure disturbance results from it. The sleep is no longer deep and restful. So these deprivation of REM sleep and of Slow wave sleep (SWS) lead to worse resting sensitiveness, morning headache, libido loss and/or impotence, concentration and decline in performance, an increased daytime sleepiness as well as one sleep attacks (KONIETZKO et al. 1993a).

7. DIAGOSTICS

The diagnosis of the obstructive sleep apnea is mainly based on two methods:

- a specific and careful case history and
- the note of the breathing during the sleep (*Polysomnonography PSG*)

The clinical OSAS symptoms are very multifaceted, very variously and partly non-specific, but they are often very characteristic, so that one must primarily close at the combination of certain symptoms on a Sleep apnea (HOCHBAN 1995).

The nightly polysomnography is, therefore the *gold standard* also that one of the Sleep apnea diagnostics for the diagnosis of all sleep disorders.

Table 8. Suitable parameters for the direct proof of SBAS
(FAUST, M. et al. 1992)

Parameters	Methods	Advantages	Disadvantages
Breathing	thermistors (mouth/nose)	small transducer, high acceptance	fixation problems; temperature drift, unless at use of a mask
	pneumotachography	exact flow and volume measuring	disturbance of the spontaneous breathing; problems of acceptance at closed system; long time calibration difficult
	induction plethysmography	separate registration thorakaler and abdomineller breath activity; Calibrating destitute of breath volumes; artefact arm	calibrating effortfully
	Measure of extension touch/pressure on-recipient	easily applying cash and very variable transducer	layer dependent sensitiveness; not calibrating cash; artefact delicate
	capnography, oxymetry	flow, O2 and CO2 measuring with a transducer	very sensitive; not calibrating cash flow
	acoustic rhinometry	quickly operably, hardly load for patients, arbitrarily often repeatable	strong dependence of lung volumes, body position and breath phase
Blood gasses	pulsoxymetry	simply applying cash; reliable and valide regulation; few movement artefacts	low sensitivity: at pO2 > 70 mmHg Apneas > 10 s still without sign. (< 4%) SaO2 waste possible
	transcutaneous pO2-measurement	high sensitivity; good indication of little fluctuations	problems of reliability; punt fluctuations of the absolute values
	transcutaneous pCO2- measurement	high sensitivity; good indication of little fluctuations	movement artefacts; heavily standardize and calibrating cash
Snoring	larynxmikro phon	small transducer; this one shows breath noise sample, sample of the different SBAS, snores	Noise artefacts (language, environment); inter individual level deviation
Heart rate	ECG; impedance ple-thysmography	standard methodology	with children and old pat. with an autonomous dysfunction no specific statement; artefacts
	measurement of non-invasive blood pressure	reliable symptom of obstructive apnea with many patients	disturbance of the sleep of a part the patients; control required (body position and decompression)

Parameters	Methods	Advantages	Disadvantages
	measurement of invasive blood pressure	reliable symptom of obstructive apnea with many patients; kontinuierl. Exact measuring	effortful invasive measuring methodology
Intrathoracal pressure differences	induction plethysmography (SIP)	specific and selectively for the obstruction of the upper respiratory tract	fixation problems; not calibrating cash; movement artefacts
	esophagus sonde	exact pressure measuring	invasive measuring method; Problems of acceptance
Body movements and body layer	actogramm	also responds to nightly Myoklonus	little specific for certain syndromes
	Finnish "mattress" (Static rank sensitive Bed)	not sleep laboratory-bound; Breathing, ECG and movement beurteibar	complicated end judging electronics
	video	easily available	time expensive, there visual evaluation

With the derivation of approx. 15 parameters the sleep can comprehensively be clarified and judged: 3 EEG channels (2 temporal, 1 occipital); 5 electrodes; 2 EOG channels ("Electrical oculography"-channels); 3 EMG channels (jaw, both legs); ECG; SaO_2; Air flow (3-pole, nose opening/mouth); breath excursions (thorax/abdomen); microphone for snoring noises; body situation; video; CPAP pressure.

Apart from the two above-mentioned methods to the diagnosis elevation there still is a whole number of special examination methods (cf. Table 8).

a) Cardiopulmonal Methods

At cardiopulmonal accompanying illnesses the health risk rises for OSAS patients considerably on, therefore a clarification is on pathologically changed cardiovascular and pulmonal functions required.

The heart circulation examinations shall clarify the being heart circulation illnesses in need of treatment like hypertonia of the small and/or great circulation, arrhythmias and insufficiency or a coronary heart disease.

At the lung function check illnesses shall more latently or more manifestly obstruction of the airways and/or a respiratorical insufficiency be stated (KONIETZKO et al. 1993a).

b) Nasopharyngeal Endoscopy

An endoscopy of the complete nose throat room is a meaningful addition for the ENT medical mirror examination. Be able to through it to establish nose corridors, made narrower polyps and pharyngeal changes, among others also symptom of a chronic vibration trauma by snoring (KONIETZKO et al. 1993a).

c) Acoustic Rhinometry

The acoustic rhinometry serves the determination of respiratory tract geometry. A defined sound wave is produced at the nose entrance. The reflection of the sound spreading is measured with a microphone.

Every variance of cross section leads into direction of propagation of the sound wave to a partial reflection. One gets the throat and nose crosscut as a function of the distance through the reflection sample recorded by the microphone of the nose entrance. Only at a standardized measuring technique one receives reliable data since the sound reflection is strongly dependent on the lung volume, the body position and the breath phase (KONIETZKO et al. 1993a, FRIDAY 1993).

d) Cephalometry

The Cephalometry (cf. Figure 6) serves the judgement craniofacial anomalies. The measuring outs of the bone and soft partial shadows in this region can be gathered from a lateral x-ray of the skull and the neck. At a sagittal shortening of the skull base sagittale shortenings of the upper and lower jaw and the skelettalen parts of the pharynx also appear.

The lower jaw itself is not abbreviated. Its retrallage is caused by a lower jaw rotation due to an abnormal vertical prolongation. The sub-face height is extended appropriately significantly. Dolichofacial face type inferring with a narrowing of the pharyngeal space on an OSAS patient so one can of a vertical (FREITAG 1993, HOCHBAN 1995).

Unless gives also *ambulant supervision methods* of the obstructive Sleep apnea to the clinical methods for the diagnosis, supervision and therapy preparation described above:

- Mesam equipment

- Pulsoxymetry
- Sleepox system and others

(RAUSCHER 1993).

8. DIFFERENTIAL DIAGNOSTICS

The conducting symptoms of the obstructive Sleep apnea are very sensitively and little specific (daytime sleepiness, snore, adiposity). Symptoms like concentration, libido loss and impotence can be put in order only with difficulty due to their ambiguity.

Putting frequent differential diagnoses of the OSAS:

- Narcolepsy
- idiopathical central nervous Hypersomnia
- periodical Hypersomnia
- alcohol and drug abuse
- early stages dementiver illnesses

(KONIETZKO et al. 1993a).

The obstructive Sleep apnea syndrome has to be delimited also of the *Prader Willi Syndrome* (DESAGA and LÄMMER 1995) and the *Obesitas Hyperventilation Syndrome* (GEIBEL et al. 1995).

9. THERAPY OF OBSTRUCTIVE SLEEP APNEA SYNDROME

The OSAS favours an increased morbidity and mortality on the one hand as a result of the Apneas even, on the other hand by the risk factors connected to it (e.g. hypertonia, arrhythmias, adiposity).

It is aim of the therapy of the OSAS to bring the breathing back to normal, to improve the symptoms like sleepiness and a one sleep inclination and to prevent a long-term progredience or subsequent illnesses or regressed it.

In the therapy you distinguish between different measures:

In the therapy one distinguishes conservative, mechanical, electrical, operative and medicinal measures.

9.1. Conservative Measures

Being part of the conservative treatment possibilities:

- weight reduction
- avoidance of alcohol and sedativa
- sleep hygiene
- sleep position training.

a) Weight Reduction

Adiposity is considered one of the main causes of the obstructive Sleep apnea syndrome, at least overweight strengthens existing breath regulation disturbances or an arrangement existing to this illness manifests, however. A weight reduction often leads to a reduction of Sleep-related breathing disturbances and to a clear improvement in the symptomatic (HOCHBAN 1995). This positive effect of the weight reduction arises from a dilatation of the pharynx due to the subcutaneous one and retropharyngeal fatty tissue reduction as well as an increasing functional residual capacity and a neuromuscular degree of effectiveness increased (KONIETZKO et al. 1993b).

b) Avoid of Alcohol and Seditiva

Small alcohol quantities (< 30 g) do not cause any change of the gas exchange and the breathing in healthy and OSAS patients. With an increasing amount of alcohol the breath drive already reduces itself significantly in the awake condition. This breath drive reduction is minted strongly particularly in old age (and in adipose people). After taking of alcohol snoring increases, the number of apneas increases and becomes the apnea duration longer (KONIETZKO et al. 1993b). Sleep and tranquillizer increase not only the daytime sleepiness, they also lead to reinforcements of the sleep-related Apneas. Till now, the extent of these side effects is not dependent on the dose predictably and not always. In interaction with other Noxen the instalment of the side effects increases (KONIETZKO et al. 1993b).

c) Sleep Hygiene

Regulated zirkadianen awake sleep rhythm can be avoided or reduced at easy illness forms sleep deficits adhere by the strict one one. A medical advice and clearing up as well as the compliance with the 10 "commandments" of an improved sleep hygiene are important:

1) Adhere to a regular day night rhythm!
2) Do not sleep longer than necessary to be had a rest after that.
3) Sleep in a cool one, room aired well!
4) Keep glaring light and disturbing noises away from your bedroom!
5) Take the last meal 2-3 hours ahead of the Zubettgehen but you do not go hungrily to bed. A glass of a warm milk can work as an easy soporific!
6) In case of one sleep difficulties light at, get up and a little calming down work!
7) Avoid chronic soporific use!
8) Exercise your body daily for 20-30 minutes!
9) Do not drink black tea, alcohol or coffee in the evening!
10) Avoid nicotine, it disturbs the sleep!

(KONIETZKO et al. 1993b).

d) Sleep Position Training

Particularly in the supine position the obstructions of the upper respiratory tract increase. This position does not favour snoring only but also the appearance probability of apneas. The pharyngeal lumen is the smallest in the supine position. It enlarges meaningfully in the side position and reaches its maximum value in sitting. In easy cases of position dependent breath disturbances an improvement can therefore be obtained by the sleep position training (KONIETZKO et al. 1993b, HOCHBAN 1995).

These methods can be at the most of use at insignificantly distinctive illnesses. So it is recommended to overweight patients in the evening to reduce their weight to renounce the alcohol and to take no soporifics and sedativa. In addition, it also is recommended to follow a regulated cirkadian awake sleep rhythm and to sleep into side position if possible since the obstructions are made easier by the supine position. In easy cases of position dependent breath disturbances an improvement can be obtained by a sleep position training.

9.2. Mechanical Measures

9.2.1. Nasal Continuous Excess Pressure Artificial Respiration (nCPAP; nBIPAP; APAP)

The *gold standard* for the treatment of the OSAS is the nightly continuous excess pressure treatment ("Continuous Positive Airway Pressure" - CPAP). The effect of the nCPAP is based on the passive pneumatic opening of the pharynx, being prevented and starting up again makes breathing times possible for a normal regular breath activity. The positive air pressure has an effect on the limitation on the side of the cavity of the abyss structures everywhere. The collapse of the upper respiratory tract can be prevented at a right attitude of the CPAP device (SULLIVAN 1981, 1989, KONIETZKO et al. 1993b, BECKER et al. 1994, BURBACH et al. 1995, BURMANN-URBANEK et al. 1995, FRIES et al. 1995 GLOSSNER-KLEISER et al. 1995a, KUHN and LUND 1995).

At the inspiration, the required pressure for the open attitude of the respiratory tract is greater than at the Exspiration. becomes in and exspiratorische pressure is regulated separated these knowledge realized and this one at the BIPAP device (on basis of the CPAP developed) (KONIETZKO et al. 1993b).

- Nasal Continous Postive AriwayPressure (nCPAP)

The effect of the nasal continuous excess pressure artificial respiration (nCPAP, nasal Continous Postive Ariway pressing aurochs) is based on the passive pneumatic string-pulling of the pharynx. The patient sleeps with a face mask made of plastic or silicone, this one with a mobile tube at an air electricity producer, here which one supplies an adjustable, easy excess pressure with the air is attached. It is demanded the patient to carry the device every night at least 4 hours.

- Biphasic positives Airway pressing aurochs-(BiPAP)

The BiPAP artificial respiration (Biphasic Positiv Airway Pressure) is comparable with that one of the CPAP artificial respiration, however with the difference that there is not only a pressure standard as in the case of the CPAP but two pressure standards which are used alternately and make so it possible that this one is exposed for patients to a higher pressure than when breathing out when breathing in with the BiPAP.

- Automatic Airway pressing aurochs (APAP)

Different methods of the automatic CPAP therapy (APAP) to the disposal which adapt to the positive printing process the current degree of obstruction the pressure customization is carried out via regular index formation (adaptationof pressure by permanent analyses of the breathing) have stood for some time. These include the breath flow, the flattening out of the inspiratorischen flow curve, snoring or measure the resistance of the upper respiratory tract directly with special oscillation technology.

9.2.2. Nasal and Oral Artificial Limbs

- Esmarch bite artificial limb

The Esmarch bite artificial limb is a synthetic material artificial limb from Paladon. The lower jaw is shifted by 3-5 mm ventrally through it. So the falling back of the tongue into the tongue reason prevented and the respiratory tract will remain open. The upper jaw teeth serve as counter-stores. The Apnoezahlen shall reduce himself and values of the partial O_2 pressure rise in the fabric, those of the partial CO_2 pressure fall, however. Morning pains in the jaw joint and Kaumuskulaturverspannungen can appear as a side effect. An effectiveness has been proved under no circumstances though (MEIER-EWERT 1989, KONIETZKO et al. 1993b, HOCHBAN 1995).

- Bite clamp

At this method the tongue is drawn with a sucking device at the lead forwards. Through this the sagittale diameter of the pharyngeal volume is extended (MATHIS 1988). The bite clamp is exclusively carried at night in which besides the lacking carrying comfort the use not proved without exception is also queried.

- Tongue vacuum protractor (ZVP)

The ZVP is a synthetic material device with a ballon clamp cavity. The tip of the tongue is told to the device into the neck in the evening. Due to the vacuum formation it gets stuck like in a neck of a bottle and is prevented so from a shift to behind.

The number and the duration of apnea phases shall be reduced. Unfortunately, it can be carried at night only 3-4 hours due to a cafing of the tongue (MEIER-EWERT 1989), in addition, its effectiveness is also extremely doubtful.

9.3. Electrical Measures

At the tongue muscle training (ZMT) a systematic electric stimulation treatment of the tongue basic musculature is carried out. Through this the muscle tonus shall be improved so that a maximum muscle atony is prevented during the sleep with transfer of the upper respiratory tract. To this end a mouth electrode shall be put under the tongue twice daily for 20-30 minutes each; a second self-adhesive electrode is fastened under the chin on the outer skin.

These two electrodes get connected to an electrical aggregate which sends out electrical impulses of low frequency and intensity for the gradual training of the tongue basic musculature in a rhythmical sequence. These current pulses shall activate the tongue basic musculature and the accompanying motor nerves and cause rhythmical muscle contract ions. However, an effective effectiveness of the ZMT could not be proved, it partly even came to a rise of the apnea hypopnea index (AHI).

9.4. Operative Measures

9.4.1. Correction of the Hindered Nose Breathing
Pharyngeal or chronically nasal obstructions of the upper respiratory tract which mainly arises due to hypertrophic tonsills are frequently the causes of snoring and the mouth breathing as well as an aggravated and irregular breathing.

With children has shown that an adenotomy and a tonsillectomy are frequently successful therapy, they can, however, reduce the complaints a little, remove under no circumstances completely, however, with the adults (MEIER-EWERT 1989).

9.4.2. Uvulo Palato Pharyngo sculpture (UPPP)
The UPPP was introduced 1981 of FUJITA et al. Sleep apnea trades itself when snoring and more easily around inter version possibility. The UPPP aims at a reduction of the soft partial fabric in the throat. Parts of the soft palate and the suppository are removed (itinerantly) under full narcosis in the hospital (UPPP) or under use of a CO_2 laser blade device. The Uvula is cut in two and shared. The number of Apneas is partly reduced, a complete cure, however, is excluded.

9.4.3. Tracheotomy
At the tracheotomy trades himself around a opening the windpipes operatively. Today, this measure seldom is only used (only into extreme situations, primarily if the patients do not cope with the CPAP treatment). It is connected to many risks and side effects so that such an operation is taken into consideration only after exclusion of all other therapy possibilities. Following the tracheotomy the obstructive apnea phases are reduced slightly and the daytime sleepiness lowered (MEIER-EWERT 1989).

9.5. Medicinal Measures

The opinions on a medicinal Schlafapanoetherapie are extremely shared. So there is no specific medicine till now, on the other hand, can be hardly predicted whether or about which medicine a patient asks. Substances mainly were breath stimulating or REM sleep supprimierender effect tested.

Some time became started *Theophyllin* at the OSAS treatment. It is a Methylxantin which has a proved stimulativen effect on the central nervous system. A complete dose up to 1000 mg/day should reduce the apnea phases (KONIETZKO et al. 1993b, HOCHBAN 1995, HEIN et al. 1995b).

Its effectiveness concerning treatment of Sleep apnea syndrome is (questionable this significant diminution of the AHI has noticed although there are some studies, however, the results of most studies contradict a symptom improvement (HEIN et al. 1993, 1995b, MEISSNER et al. 1995).

Nicotine is discussed as a therapy suggestion in the newer literature, although the number of Apneas reduced itself during the first two sleep hours but the result nevertheless was not significant (HEIN et al. 1995a).

Chapter 4

THE OBSTRUCTIVE SLEEP APNEA SYNDROME AS A RISK FACTOR PHYSICAL DISEASEES

The role of the obstructive Sleep apnea syndrome as a cause of cardiovascular diseasees are frequently discussed (PETER and PODSZUS 1993; WOLK et al 2003 b, LAVIE P. 2004, SVATIKOVA et al. 2005, LAVIE L. and LAVIE P. 2006).

SCHÄFER et al. (1998) as well as KIELY and McNICHOLAS (2000) refer, however, for cardiovascular diseasees in OSAS patients to the anyway high risk profile so that a causal connection cannot be derived absolutely from these correlations.

But already 1976 described TILKIAN et al. an arterial blood rise in pressure in OSAS patients. This OSAS conditional hypertonus was repeated found also by many other authors in the following period (e.g. PODSZUS 1988, EHLENZ et al. 1991, BIXLER et al. 2000, SCHNEIDER et al. 2000, WOLK et al. 2003a). Bixler et al. found a correlation of the blood pressure values with the height of the RDI index which got weaker however with an advancing age of the patients concerned. Schneider et al. found pulmonary arterial increased in these patients furthermore pressure values. STEINER and STRAUER (2004) described an available nightly pulmonary arterial hypertonia with the 20 percent risk of one also developing hypertonia on the day persistierende pulmonary arterial. As causes the Euler-Liljestrand reflex and the Remodeling mechanisms for the persistency are mentioned for these nightly rises in pressure on the day.

An increased prevalence of the obstructive Sleep apnea syndrome was described also for the coronary heart disease (De OLAZABAL et al. 1982, KÖHLER and SCHÄFER 1996, SANNER et al. 1996), partial the OSAS got named as an independent risk factor also here (DUCHNA et al. 2001, WOLK and SOMERS 2003).

CHEN und SCHARF could prove 1998 hypokinesias of the dependent myocard during apnea phases in sedated pigs with stenoses of the Ramus interventricularis anterior, what could be explain this repeatedly described increased risk of mortality in OSAS patients with a coronary heart disease (PODSZUS 1988, SCHÄFER et al. 1998, LAVIE L. 2004) or the risk cardial events of these patients (SCHÄFER et al. 1999) and the progressing of the coronary heart disease (WOLK and SOMERS 2003).

Both ANDREAS et al. (1991) and HANLY et al. (1993) found during obstructive apneas elektrocardiographical increases ST way reductions lasting, also in patients with negative ergometric. So how far these ECG changes can actually be ascribed to myocardial ischemias is, however, still unclear.

NAKAMURA et al. (2004) described a QT dispersion in OSA patients, what an increased arrhythmia inclination implies. TILKIAN et al. (1977) actually watched sinusbradycardias with asystolias up to 6.3 seconds, intermittent AV blockings II. degree as well as a self-limiting ventricular tachycardia.

In addition, the authors who (see above) examined the cardiovascular risk factors found an increased prevalence of the peripheral arterial seal disease (leg providing vessels).

Furthermore largely correspondingly are described about a high prevalence of the obstructive Sleep apnea syndrome at cerebrovascular events (ischemic seizure/stroke, transient ischemic attack TIA) (BASSETTI and ALDRICH 1999, NACHTMANN et al. 2003, MOHSENIN 2004, YAGGI and MOHSENIN 2004, LAVIE L. 2005, LAVIE L. and LAVIE P. 2006).

Only few authors contradict these results (MERRITT 2004). According to Cadilhac and Thorpe, it can come in the first six months after a cerebrovascular seizure to a spontaneous improvement in the OSAS (CADILHAC et al. 2005).

General could be proved in OSAS patients a serological cardiovascular risk factors like increased homocysteine mirrors due to the formation of free radicals at endothelial dysfunction (LAVIE et al. 2001, SVATIKOVA et al. 2004, LAVIE L. and LAVIE P. 2004, LAVIE L. and LAVIE P. 2005a and b) and an increased coaguability (von KANEL and DIMSDALE 2003, PARISH and SOMERS 2004), so that an increased risk for cardiovascular events generally and due to a swelling of the vessel wall of the Arteria carotis for cerebrale ischemias in particular is accepted by these authors (CLARENBACH and WESSENDORF 2001, SILVESTRINI et al. 2002). FRANKLIN (2002) describes furthermore still malicious dynamic fluctuations during and in completion of an obstructive apnea as a trigger cerebrovascular events. So not only the coincidence is described to events but the OSAS as an independent risk factor named for these events by OSAS and cerebrovascular often (NEAU 2001, DIAZ and SEMPERE 2004).

In addition, the obstructive Sleep apnea syndrome increases the insulin resistance (HARSCH et al. 2004a and b) and therefore leads to a disturbed glucose metabolism in patients with diabetics (MESLIER et al. 2003), i.e. it worsens a preexistent Diabetes mellitus. COUGHLIN et al. (2004) describe the OSAS as a risk factor for the metabolic syndrome.

ARRUDA-OLSON et al. (2003) point to the risk of the development of an erectile dysfunction. NEAU et al. (2002) regard the obstructive Sleep apnea syndrome as risk factor for headaches, YANTIS (1999) and BÜTTNER and RÜHLE (2004d) also regard it as a risk factor for depressions.

Chapter 5

DAYTIME SYMPTOMATICS AT OSAS

1. ATTENTION PROCESSES AND EXCESSIVE DAYTIME SLEEPINESS (EDS) IN SLEEP APNEA PATIENTS

1.1. General

In addition, at many sleep-related diseases, among others Hypersomnias and Dyssomnias, the persons affected suffer nightly symptomatic besides hers under increased daytime sleepiness and one a sleep inclination (BÜTTNER et al. 2004e). In turn these are accompanied by attention-related deficits and a qualified sense (GERDESMEYER et al. 1997, MÜLLER et al. 1997, RANDERATH et al. 1997, 1998, WEESS 1997, WEESS et al. 1998, BÜTTNER et al. 2003b, 2004c).

An increased accident danger at work as well as in the traffic and therefore a social medical risk increased are among others result of this reduced physical fitness (e.g. BRADLEY et al. 1985, PODSZUS et al. 1986, HE et al. 1988, MITTLER et al. 1988, LAMPHERE et al. 1989, ROEHRS et al. 1989, BÉDARD et al. 1991, KRIBBS et al. 1993, GERDESMEYER et al. 1997, RANDERATH et al. 1997, 1998, WEESS 1997, WEESS et al. 1998, BÜTTNER et al. 2000a and b, BÜTTNER 2001).

The difficulty of investigating the connection between sleep, daytime sleepiness and physical fitness as well as mental fitness is mainly based on three conditions (JOHNSON 1982, WEESS 1997, WEESS et al. 1998). So becoming the three above-mentioned parameters by a variety of other variables influenced, e.g. by the motivation of the experimentee or patient or the day rhythmic or the week rhythmic. Furthermore the daytime sleepiness and the fitness represent both and the attention conditional processes underlying them complex constructs. In addition, this analysis makes more difficult for concept uses by lack more uniformly terms in the medical and psychological literature (JOHNSON 1982, WEESS 1997, WEESS et al. 1998).

A number of miscellaneous research approaches and definitions exists in the medical and therefore also in the sleep medical research regarding the attention as well as attention controlled processes (RÜTZEL 1977, RAPP 1982, BRICKENKAMP and KARL 1986, POSNER and RAFAL 1987, SÄRING 1988, POSNER and PETERSEN 1990, POSNER 1995), just like already described under I. 1., which respectively elevate other qualities and aspects of the fitness during the day (JAMES 1890, HEAD 1926, MACKWORTH, J.F. 1956, MACKWORTH, N. 1958, SCHMIDTKE 1965, NORMAN 1973, BÄUMLER 1974, HARNATT 1975, RÜTZEL 1977, BRICKENKAMP and KARL 1986, POSNER and RAFAL 1987, SÄRING 1988, POSNER and PETERSEN 1990, ROLLET 1993, SCHÖTTKE and WIEDL 1993).

The concept of Posner and Rafal (1987) is mainly used in the sleep medical literature (KELLER et al. 1993, WEESS 1997, WEESS et al. 1998).

In addition, the empirical recording of the attention and its components carried out very miscellaneously as well as the different quality of validity of the employed methods and of testing instruments are problematic.

So among others the vigilance measured by means of unsuitable test requirements (STEPHEN et al. 1991), too complex test requirements (BÉDARD et al. 1893) or too shortly test requirements (BÉDARD et al. 1991, 1993, WEESS 1997, WEESS et al. 1998).

For the recording of the one sleep inclination at an obstructive Sleep apnea syndrome the MSLT (Multiple Sleep Latency Test) is carried out today mostly (POCETA et al. 1992), since it correlates with the subjective state of the OSAS most strongly. DENZEL et al. becomes (the attention or the vigilance grasped at the most indirectly through it, though 1993).

According to this end Denzel et al. (1993) searched and in connection with this two computer-controlled neuropsychological methods of testing, a vigilance and an attention test how the latter was checked among three trial conditions (visually, acoustically and combined), examined according to more suitable methods. Significant differences found themselves before and after a nCPAP therapy at the testung at both tasks (*dual task* and *vigilance*) (DENZEL et al. 1993).

Similar results, i.e. a clear improvement in the vigilance under nCPAP already also found SCHWARZENBERGER-KESPER et al. (1991) and CASSEL et al. (1991).

The standardization of the trial conditions also proved to be meaningful (HORN et al. 1983, DENZEL et al. 1993) as well as the conception test setup (author).

It shown, that an immediate acoustic feedback improved the motivation of the patients about the correctness of the reactions having been carried out and covered the consequences of the sleep deprivation and the performance losses resulting from it up by which (WILKINSON 1961, STEYVERS and GAILLARD 1993, WEESS 1997, WEESS et al. 1998).

1.2. Daytime Sleepiness, a One Sleep Inclination and Road Performance

1.2.1. The Connection between Obstructive Sleep Apnea and Risk of Accident

Many people complain about "permanent sleepiness" or "chronic exhaustion"; the prevalence of this symptom in the population is valued at 20% (BATES et al. 1993). There undoubtedly are fluent transitions between more distinctively, however (e.g. after a period of intensive effort) still "normal" sleepiness and conditions of diseased fatigue. A source of misunderstandings and diagnostic miscarriages of justice is the ambiguity of the German concept "sleepiness" by which quite different physical and emotional conditions are marked. In the narrower, real meaning of the word "tiredness" stands for "sleepiness": a condition of increased one sleep readiness. However, with "tiredness" a condition gets (predominating in the musculature noticeable) also more general exhaustion marks after physical efforts; this must be not at all accompanied by sleep inclination. Furthermore the same concept is used for a physical exhaustion without a clear relation to preceded efforts, a state for which the word would rather be "buggering" at the place. Frequently accompany or result of physical diseasees for example of infections is such a form of the "tiredness". Gives fluent transitions predominantly to the conditions from here to spiritual "exhaustion" which disturbances have more emotionally subsumed for themselves under different categories. It is quite decisive for a clear diagnosis position in "chronic tiredness" to differentiate here linguistical at first and to get a clear idea of this what the patient exactly means if he speaks about "tiredness".

The decisive diagnostic course is the question how far the "chronic tiredness" of the patient represents a genuine *Hypersomnia*. A Hypersomnia according to the psychiatric and sleep medical classification systems (DSM-IV, American Psychiatric Association 1994; ICSD, American Sleep Disorders Association

1990) is defined as an excessive sleepiness during the day; this can shown himself by prolonged night sleep episodes, by a permanent sleep need during the day and/or by the regular appearance of either one or several day sleep episodes (in the extreme case spontaneous in the form of "sleep attacks").

The ability to lead a vehicle surely and accident-freely needs a certain degree of sustained attention and alertness GUILLEMINAULT et al. (GUILLEMINAULT et al. 1978, BRADLEY et al. 1985, PODSZUS et al. 1986, FINDLEY et al. 1988a, 1988b, 1989b, 1990, 1991, 1995, HE et al. 1988, MITLER et al. 1988, LAMPHERE et al. 1989, ROEHRS et al. 1989, BÉDARD et al. 1991, CASSEL et al. 1991a, 1991b, 1993, 1996, KRIBBS et al. 1993, ATS 1994, MARTIN et al. 1996, GERDESMEYER et al. 1997, KRIEGER et al. 1997, RANDERATH et al. 1997, 1998, WEESS 1997, WEESS et al. 1998, BÜTTNER et al. 2000a and b, BÜTTNER 2001).

As a rule, a cut-rate sustained attention and vigilance and/or an increased sleepiness or one sleep inclination draw an affected reaction readiness and reaction ability as well as an accident inclination increased after themselves (the above-mentioned authors).

Reliable details or numbers about attention conditional causes of an accident are not available due to the German data protection definitions. According to Seko et al. (1986) 45% of all fatal traffic accidents became caused, loudly a so-called second sleep 1986 detail of the Statistical Federal Office Wiesbaden (1988) however only 0.5% of all road accidents through falling asleep at the steering wheel or this one (SEKO et al. 1986, Statistical Federal Office Wiesbaden 1988, CASSEL et al. 1993).

A study of Zulley et al. (1995) showed that 38% of all road accidents can be explained by a reduced vigilance on Bavarian motorways; when the most frequent individual cause yielded at this with 24% of all serious accidents the drop off or himself sleeps at the steering wheel (ZULLEY et al. 1995)

These sleep conditional vigilance or sustained attention reductions were primarily (still strengthened by the effect of the biological rhythmic (HILDEBRANDT et al. 1974, HILDEBRANDT 1976, MITLER 1991, CASSEL et al. 1991c, 1993, ZULLEY 1995).

Already 1955 Prokop and Prokop discussed the meaning of fatigue and a one sleep inclination regarding the roadworthiness – though without research of sleep disorder caused aspects or causes (PROKOP and PROKOP 1955, CASSEL et al. 1993).

But only 1978 Guilleminault et al. pointed out a risk increased perhaps for patients with Sleep-related breath disturbances (GUILLEMINAULT et al. 1978, CASSEL et al. 1991a, 1991b).

George et al. (1987) took up this assumption and examined the accident probability of 27 suspected OSAS patients. With 93% of the patients the Motor Vehicle Branch of Manitoba (Canada) was accidents listed in the accident register but only in 54% of the control group participants. Unfortunately, the polysomnographic confirmation of the suspicion diagnosis as well as the details on the time period of the given accidents are missing among seven patients (GEORGE et al. 1987, CASSEL et al. 1991a, 1991b, WEESS 1997, WEESS et al. 1998).

Findley et al. (1988b) found an accident probability increased three times at 29 OSAS patients (AHI > 5) opposite all driving licence owners of Virginia (USA) and even one increased seven foldly opposite a control group (n = 35). Findley et al. did not indicate whether the OSAS diagnosis was already known to the interview (FINDLEY et al. 1988b, CASSEL et al. 1991a, 1991b, WEESS 1997, WEESS et al. 1998).

Later studies and examinations of Cassel et al. (1991a, 1991b, 1996), of ATS (1994) and of Krieger et al. (1997) confirmed these results. So seem to patients to suffer from distinctive sleepiness and second sleep in a Sleep apnea syndrome strengthened during the driving (cf. also George et al. 1987, FINDLEY et al. 1988b). With an increasing impairment of the persons affected by the symptomatic of the obstructive Sleep apnea the self-caused sustained attention conditional accidents also occurred increasingly (CASSEL et al. 1991a, 1991b, 1996, ATS 1994, KRIEGER et al. 1997).

1.2.2. Recording of the Vigilance and the Sustained Attention at Obstructive Sleep Apnea Syndrome (OSAS)

Reduced sustained attention and daytime sleepiness increased therefore represent an increased risk of accident at an obstructive Sleep apnea syndrome. So can be limited both the driving ability and the fitness for work of the persons affected considerably (WEESS 1997, WEESS et al. 1998).

Aldrich et al. (1992) could shown, that during the day 71% of the accidents from 424 sleep disturbed patients rise by extreme sleepiness (due to experimental examinations) and that the severity degree of the disease had an essential influence (Aldrich 1992, WEESS 1997, WEESS et al. 1998). George et al. found an increased risk of accident even at 93% of the OSAS patients (GEORGE et al. 1997, CASSEL et al. 1991a, 1991b, WEESS 1997, WEESS et al. 1998). Findley et al. (1988b) calculated one increased risk three till seven foldly (FINDLEY et al. 1988b, CASSEL 1991a, 1991b, WEESS 1997, WEESS et al. 1998).

Under nCPAP therapy thre is a clear fall in the daytime sleepiness visible already after short time, which it is recording mostly with the Multiple Sleep

Latency Test MSLT (CARSCADON et al. 1986) and the Maintenance of Wakefulness Test MWT (POCETA et al. 1992).

While the MSLT is grasping the one sleep latency in monotonous situations, the ability to remain awake is measured and objectified with the MWT. The latter therefore gets professional requirements at all sorts of clinical questions used, particularly to the judgement of the fitness to drive and more especially (GERDESMEYER et al. 1997).

Both the MSLT and the MWT measure the alertness stage in terms of there Walsleben (1992) examined whether both also include the watchfulness ("alertness") or whether the measured alertness stage of the vigilance corresponds. Since this is not the case examination methods had to be sought, which more adequately examines the sustained attention or the vigilance (WALSLEBEN 1992, RANDERATH et al. 1997).

For some time driving simulation programmes have therefore been used more and more to grasp vigilance and sustained attention deficits in patients with an obstructive Sleep apnea syndrome (author).

So Findleys working group 1989 introduced a driving simulator (Steer Clear) for the recording of the fitness to drive from OSAS patients, a monotonous driving situation is represented and obstacles must be gone round (FINDLEY et al. 1989b).

Findley et al. could prove, that patients with an obstructive Sleep apnea obtained considerably worse test results (approx. triple mistake rate) than the persons of the control group and that unfavourable test results yielded correlations with a high accident instalment (FINDLEY et al. 1988b, 1989a, 1989b, 1990, 1991, 1995, CASSEL et al. 1991b, GERDESMEYER et al. 1997, RANDERATH et al. 1997).

At an examination before and to nCPAP therapy a clear recovery of the mistake rate (50 per cent diminution) could be established after a 3- to 5-month therapy at the Steer Clear (FINDLEY et al. 1989a, GERDESMEYER et al. 1997, RANDERATH et al. 1997).

In the consequence different driving simulators became developed, among others the DADT (Divided Attention Driving Test) of George et al., which should include the multimodal construction of the complex car road performance (GEORGE et al. 1996a, 1996b, 1997, RANDERATH et al. 1997). The DADT is based on Moscowitz (1977) test to the diveded attention (MOSCOWITZ et al. 1977). A position indicator shall be formed of an aim box by tracking (GEORGE et al. 1996, 1996b). Cassel et al. used a 80-minute sustained attention test, however, to prove nCPAP effects (CASSEL et al. 1996).

The driving simulator test "CARDA" (Ambrocker vigilance test) which shall include the degree of vigilance was developed in the Ambrocker working group in 1997. It is based on the principles of the Steer Clear of Findley et al. (1989b). The driving simulator test "CARSIM" was developed in the Ambrocker working group in 1998. It based on the principles of the DADT of George et al. (1996a, 1996b, 1997); but it is a consequent further development. Both at CARDA (GERDESMEYER et al. 1997, RANDERATH et al. 1997, 1998, 2000) and at CARSIM (BÜTTNER et al. 2000a and b, BÜTTNER 2001) pretherapeutical found themselves a considerably higher mistake rate than under nCPAP therapy and opposite a control group.

2. MEMORY PROCESSES AND COGNITIVE FITNESS IN SLEEP APNEA PATIENTS

2.1. General

Studying tasks which are presented before a sleep phase or period are kept better than these, these are presented before an awake period. This could for the first time experimentally be proved by JENKINS and DALLENBACH (1924). This effect favouring the memory is covered by many experimental examinations (SMITH 1996, HENNEVIN et al. 1995). With the discovery of the REM sleep (DEMENT and KLEITMAN 1957) the starting signal fell for a more specific research programme by special roles being assigned to respectively certain sleep stadia for the memory processes. In the consequence got on the one hand the REM sleep, among other things due to its special physiological changes, effects memory favouring also ascribed to the Slow-Wave Sleep (SWS) on the other hand, however (HOBSON and McCARLEY 1977, CRICK 1983, SQUIRE and ALVAREZ 1995, WILSON and McNAUGHTON 1994, KARNI et al. 1994).

Diseasees have also considerable consequences sleep drawee besides the nightly symptomatic on the day. So an excessive daytime sleepiness appears as a main symptom of the OSAS with a partly imperative sleep impulse. It assume, that reduced sleep quality to be frequently found this one at sleep disorders lead to a reduced relaxation function of the night sleep because of deep sleep or REM suppression, increased nightly Arousal reactions or awake phases extended (WEESS et al. 1998). According to JENNUM et al. (1993), Insomnia and sleepiness influence the cognitive functions. Patients with problems of excessive daytime sleepiness have special problems in situations of physical quiet and at for a long time continual monotonous concentration tasks (SCHWARZENBERGER-KESPER et al. 1987).

In a study of KALES (1985) 76% of the OSAS patients show cognitive deficits in the areas of thinking, on-capacity, memory, communication and the ability to learn new information. NAËGELÉ et al. (1995) examined different cognitive functions in Sleep apnea patients. They found out that OSAS patients were impaired at executive functions which contain the acquisition of information for the memory processing. CASSEL et al. (1989) could state a reduced cognitive non verbal performance and processing speed in Sleep apnea patients. They could prove a degraded cognitive processing speed in OSAS patients in the Number Connection Test ZVT[1]. KOTTERBA et al. (1998) found an impairment of the central nervous activation (alertness), the selective attention and the sustained attention in OSAS patients. In another examination of Kotterba et al. (1997) 32 of 40 OSAS patients showed pathological results in the ZVT. Also pathological results and a normalization under nCPAP found BÜTTNER et al. (2003a and b) in 50 OSAS patients both in the ZVT and in the Benton test[2] (= post pathological intelligence). BARBÉ et al. (1998) and BÜTTNER et al. (2003b, 2004c) proved in Sleep apnea patients a reduced vigilance.

Accidents or "almost accidents" were result of impaired fitness due to sleepiness and lack of sleep in OSAS patients in the traffic or at work. Different studies themselves let be seen, that patients who suffers from a Sleep apnea syndrome show a risk of accident increased strongly in comparison with norm collectives and represent a relevant dangerous driving for himself and other participants (ALDRICH et al.1989, CASSEL et al. 1991, FINDLEY et al. 1991, 2000, BARBÉ et al. 1998, TERÁN-SANTOS et al. 1999, HORSTMANN et al. 2000).

George et al. (1999) examined the accident instalments and the number of traffic offences of OSAS patients with the result that the accident frequency and the number of traffic violations were increased in comparison with a control group during a period from five years. According to Young et al. (1997) the relative risk of causing an accident within 5 years is increased by the factor 3 for men with a Sleep-related breathing disturbance. Several examinations cover one around 2- to 3-fold, up to 7-fold increased risk of accident (George et al. 1987, 1999 FINDLEY et al. 1988, 2000).

In connection with this, professional drivers, bus and heavy goods vehicle drivers represent a special group since they spend professionally much time in the

---

[1] ZVT = Zahlen-Verbindungs-Test (english: Number Connection Test; OSWALD & ROTH 1987); measured: cognitive processing speed
[2] Benton-Test (BENTON 1974); measured: post pathological intelligence

street and moreover drive as a rule bigger vehicles with partly dangerous cargo load or other persons so that in the case of an accident probably more considerable damages and injuries can occur. These persons have way of life connected with that by their profession and this an increased risk of falling ill with disturbances with an OSAS. So truck drivers have e.g. a very irregular sleep awake rhythm (STRADLING 1989, STOOHS et al. 1995). In 1994 STOOHS et al. examined the influence of Sleep-related breathing disturbances (SBAS) and adiposity with commercial drivers of big lorry trailers. Drivers with SBAS cause twice as many accidents per driven 1000 miles, as which without SBAS, how the adiposity still increased the accident instalment. Accidents caused by oversleepiness conditional driving incapableness/ incompetency and criminal offences connected with that should have accepted an extent under professional strength driving which is comparable with the drunkenness crime (MEYER 1990).

2.2. Causes Neuropsychological Deficits

In the literature the pathophysiological connections of neuropsychological deficits are discussed controversially at an obstructive Sleep apnea syndrome. Two concepts are favoured predominantly. On the one hand, the nightly hypoxies and on the other hand the disturbed sleep architecture for neuropsychological or cognitive deficits are held responsible.

However, a clear separation of both factors is hardly possible at the OSAS since both conditions appear together here, as a rule. Different studies illustrate a connection between nightly oxygen desaturation and different neuropsychological or cognitive parameters. So seeing Greenberg et al. (1987) the nightly hypoxies as a cause of the neuropsychological deficits and the daytime sleepiness. In an examination of FINDLEY et al. (1986) however, the hypoxies do correlate with the degree of the cognitive impairment, but not with the sleep fragmentation during the sleep and awake phases.

MONTPLAISIR et al. (1992) see the best forecast factor in the nightly hypoxies both for the alertness on the day and for the daytime sleepiness. In a study of KOTTERBA et al. (1998) different neuropsychological parameters correlate with the degree of the hypoxies, but not with the Arousal index and the AHI.

Other examinations see the reason for the neuropsychological deficits and particularly for the daytime sleepiness rather in the disturbance of the sleep architecture according to a sleep fragmentation, thorough with a diminution of the REM sleep and deep sleep share (Slow wave sleep). So rejected BONNET et al.

(1985) after, that a sleep fragmentation already leads to neuropsychological impairments in healthies. GUILLEMINAULT et al. (1988) could not establish relation between the daytime sleepiness and respiratorical parameters like the RDI or the oxygen desaturation in a study in OSAS patients. They rather saw the best predictor in the sleep fragmentation for the markedness of the day sleepiness. Also TELAKIVI et al. (1988) ascribe the neuropsychological deficits a greater importance – to cause the Sleep fragmentation. This is supported by the results of COLT et al. (1991). In this examination nightly hypoxies which did not perform influence on the daytime sleepiness were induced under CPAP-Theapie at a normal sleep architecture during a night. They concluded, that the intermittent decrease of the nightly oxygen repletion does not lead to increased daytime sleepiness into absence from sleep fragmentation.

According to BÉDARD et al. (1991) a multifaktorielles event is the most probable, at which both the sleep fragmentation and the nightly hypoxies reduced vigilance or neuropsychological deficits lead in which the hypoxies seem to play a larger role in servere cases.

The daytime sleepiness made responsibly even for the cognitive deficits also gets additional (ROEHRS et al. 1995). In turn other examinations see neither in disturbed sleep architecture nor in the nightly hypoxies a reason for the neuropsychological deficits in OSAS patients.

So could for Ingram et al. (1994) no differences with regard to the vigilance between OSAS patients and norm experimentees establish. The vigilance rather reduced itself with an advancing age. Examinations of KOTTERBA et al. (1998) and BÜTTNER et al. (2004c) prove, however, the opposite. They found differences of the vigilance, however no age differences, between OSAS patients and healthies.

Perhaps the severity degree of the OSAS or the CPAP-Compliance also plays a role, measured with the AHI or the RDI, (CASSEL et al. 1989, ENGLEMAN et al. 1993, JOHNS et al. 1993).

3. DISCUSSION OF THE RESULTS

The obstructive Sleep apnea syndrome impairs the patients concerned considerably besides the nightly symptomatic also on the day. It can be named the excessive daytime sleepiness as well as performance impairments as cardinal symptoms on the day (WEESS et al. 1998). Neuropsychological and cognitive deficits could be proved in OSAS patients in different studies (Bédard et al. 1991, Naëgelé et al. 1995, Gresele et al. 1996, Engleman et al. 2000, BÜTTNER et al.

2003a and b). As a reason for these deficits different factors are held responsible. So on the one hand the nightly hypoxies and on the other hand also disturbed sleep architecture can lead to a distinctive daytime sleepiness.

Cognitive Differences between Patients with Obstructive Sleep Apnea Syndrome and Healthies

As already mentioned above, patients who suffer from a Sleep apnea syndrome are impaired besides the nightly symptomatic also on the day. So have to be called the excessive daytime sleepiness as well as performance impairments as cardinal symptoms during the day (Weeß et al., 1998). In addition, neuropsychological and cognitive deficits could be proved in OSAS patients in several studies (BÉDARD et al. 1991, NAËGELÉ et al. 1995, GRESELE et al. 1996, ENGLEMAN et al., 2000, BÜTTNER et al. 2003a and b).

In the examination of BÜTTNER et al. (2003a and b) the OSAS patients (n = 50) came off in comparison with healthies ones in the non verbal intelligence test for the recording of the cognitive processing and performance speed (Number Connection Test: ZVT) statistically significantly worse. CASSEL et al. (1989) also could prove a degraded cognitive processing speed in OSAS patients in the ZVT. In an examination of KOTTERBA et al. (1997) 32 of 40 OSAS patients showed pathological results in the ZVT.

In the Benton test for the recording of the fitness of the visual noticing ability the OSAS patients showed significantly worse results only with regard to the number of mistakes, compared with healthies. At number of correct accounts differences concerning the mean average values and standard deviations between OSAS patients and healthies also found themselves, without being statistically relevant, however (BÜTTNER et al. 2003a and b).

Last one could on the one hand envelop duly be on the sample composition or this complexity. The increased number of mistakes and the simultaneously almost normal number of correct answers also could on the other hand represent a criterion or characteristic for the recording neurocognitive deficit at OSAS-Paienten, however.

Result
It can be said that OSAS patients are different from healthies regarding cognitive skills. This outer himself both in the memory processes (Benton test) and in the cognitive processing and performance speed (ZVT). These impairments can have a serious consequences if or as long as they remain untreated.

CPAP Therapy and Its Effect

In the examination of BÜTTNER et al. (2003a and b) it came already after a 3-day nCPAP therapy for a clear improvement in the fitness of the visual noticing ability (Benton test) and in the cognitive information processing speed (ZVT). These results are supported by other studies. It was thought so that a significant improvement which increased after 42 days again and shows according to tendency better values in comparison with the norm collective already let itself be seen after 2 nights nCPAP therapy in OSAS patients in the ZVT.

Improved performances could be established at driving simulator examinations under nCPAP therapy in different other studies. So patients pointed in an examination of RANDERATH et al. (1997) already after a night with an optimal print alignment a significant reduction of the error rate. Will not clearly whether this result cannot be explained by a learning effect due to the short time period between the testung before and under the therapy, though. George et al. (1997) and FINDLEY et al. (1989) come with the DADT or the Steer-Clear test as well as later BÜTTNER et al. (1999b) after examinations also to the result, that the vigilance, attention or there performances can be improved under CPAP therapy.

Also in the real situations the road accident instalment is reduced by the machine-aided therapy. So CASSEL and employees (1996) watched one in OSAS patients reduction of the accident instalment under nCPAP therapy from 0.8/100000 km to 0.15/100000 km.

With regard to the change of the neuropsychological parameters or test performances under CPAP therapy there exists knowledge following in the scientific literature till now:

So a reduction could be proved of both the subjective and the objective daytime sleepiness in several studies (MONTPLAISIR et al. 1992, ENGLEMAN et al. 1993, 1994, DOUGLAS et al. 2000). According to SCHWARZENBERGER-KESPER et al. (1987), the improvement in the daytime sleepiness is an essential motive for a good therapy compliance of the patients. SFORZA and LUGARESI (1995) stated a reduced objective daytime sleepiness after a one-year nCPAP therapy, this one, however, prepare therapy interruption after a night again himself increased. In addition, a recovery of the neuropsychological deficits could be verified in several studies. KOTTERBA et al. (1998) found, that the divided attention as well as the cognitive performance and processing speed rejected a significant improvement both the simple after. Lamphere et al. (1989) proved already after a therapy night a significant improvement in the attention this one nCPAP brought itself back to normal after 14 days. An improvement in the vigilance or the sustained attention and different cognitive deficits due to the nCPAP therapy were also described repeatedly (DENZEL et al. 1993, ENGLEMAN et al. 1994, RANDERATH 1997, 2000, BÜTTNER 1999b).

Other examinations arose, however, that himself the cognitive one and neuropsychological deficits not or only in sections improve, what could point out to an irreversible hypoxic damage of the ZNS (MONTPLAISIR et al. 1992, BÉDARD et al. 1993, KOTTERBA et al. 1998) and the importance of an early diagnosis and therapy of the OSAS therefore underlines.

During the day, the daytime sleepiness reduced, vigilance and attention could be increased by means of additional offering of Theophylline in patients who suffered from this residual symptomatic (BÜTTNER and RÜHLE 2003a, 2004a).

Result

The difference or the improvement after an effective nCPAP therapy speaks consequences the sleep for the necessity to use this therapy in OSAS patients concerned to possibly avoid serious impairments at the memory processes or in the cognitive fitness or make this one possible for patients no more under the during the day appearing suffer have to Sleep apnea syndrome.

Influence of the Vigilance and Daytime Sleepiness on the Memory Processes or the Cognitive Fitness

Increased daytime sleepiness is one of the most frequent reasons for road accidents. Sleepiness at the steering wheel is in up to 25% of the triggers of motorway accidents (LANGLOIS et al. 1985, PAKOLA et al. 1995, HORNE and REYNER 1995). An examination of 67671 car accidents not caused by alcohol in France within the years 1994-1998 showed that the risk is increased significantly for accidents with death consequence and with heavy injuries at sleepiness-related accidents in comparison with not sleepiness-related accidents (PHILIP and MITLER 2000). An analysis of the fatal accidents on Bavarian motorways in the year 1991 pointed, that 49 of 204 accidents (24%) was triggered by falling asleep at the steering wheel (DANNER and LANGWIEDER 1994). In turn the obstructive Sleep apnea syndrome represents one of the most frequent reasons for the increased daytime sleepiness (AMERICAN THORACIC SOCIETY 1994, McNICHOLAS 1999). So several studies pointed that patients with an OSAS one up to have risk of accident increased 7 times in comparison with healthies (GEORGE et al. 1987, FINDLEY et al. 1988, FINDLEY et al. 1991, YOUNG et al. 1997, BARBÉ et al. 1998, TERÁN-SANTOS et al. 1999, HORSTMANN et al. 2000).

Even with patients who did not show the full frame of an OSAS yet there was already a distinctive daytime sleepiness and therefore a risk of accident increased.

According to YOUNG et al. (1997) the relative risk is increased by the factor 3 at habitual or heavy snorers to cause an accident within 5 years. The danger of falling asleep unintentionally at patients with OSAS still is strengthened in subjectively felt monotonous situations (CASSEL et al. 1991). It is to consider that all patients who have fallen ill with an OSAS do not show an increased risk of accident by se (GEORGE 2000), though. Falling asleep at the steering wheel is not the only explanation reason for accidents either. It has to be taken into account that tired persons also frequently cause accidents without having fallen asleep actually (GEORGE 2000). Attention faults and a reduced discernment seem rather to cause an increased accident frequency due to the sleepiness (PHILIP and MITLER 2000).

Till now, it was not examined, whether and how the daytime sleepiness and the vigilance influenced the memory processes or the cognitive fitness. To get clean findings and be able to interpret the found neurocognitive impairments correctly, a possible connection of these two factors (daytime sleepiness and vigilance) with the results of the Benton test and those of the ZVTs had to be excluded.

In my examination no meaningful connections between these two factors and the cognitive parameters could be found so that the found results of the OSAS patients with Benton test and with the ZVT can be explained by the symptomatic of the Sleep apnea syndrome. This could have taken place, because other factors could be participated at the memory processes than at the vigilance and the daytime sleepiness.

Result
Since in my examination no significant connection between the daytime sleepiness and the vigilance and the neurocognitive processes (Benton test, ZVT) could be found at the OSAS patients, these deficits could be explained by the processes of this disease taking place at night.

Severity Degree of the Disease
Up till now only the influence of the severity degree of an OSAS on the accident frequency or the risk of accident was examined. Measured so some examinations yielded a connection between the severity degree of the disease with the AHI or RDI and the accident inclination increased (ALDRICH 1989, CASSEL et al. 1991, ALPERT et al. 1992, TERÁN-SANTOS et al. 1999, HORSTMANN et al. 2000). BARBÉ et al. (1998) and YOUNG et al. (1997)

could prove, however, that in OSAS patients, although the risk of accident is increased, it does not depend on the severity degree of the disease. GEORGE et al. (1999) concluded in an examination, that only patients with a severe OSAS with an AHI > 40 have increased car accidents.

In my examination no connections also arose between the fitness of the visual noticing ability (Benton test), the cognitive information processing speed (ZVT) and the severity degree of the disease. From this is to conclude, that persons affected show the same cognitive impairments both easily and heavily.

On the one hand, these neuropsychological or cognitive deficits could be explained by the nightly hypoxies and also disrupted sleep architecture on these on the other hand (are primarily the deep sleep stadia / Slow wave sleep which play a decisive role in the memory formation and the processes reduced).

Result

Is the treatment of the Sleep apnea syndrome absolutely requiredly, independent of the severity degree, there the cognitive or memory performances of all persons affected show deficits. To avoid underestimation of the disease you must point out that all patients suffering from an OSAS are in need of treatment. This treatment would help the ailing ones to reduce the results of the OSAS (among others cognitive and memory deficits).

Chapter 6

QUALITY OF LIFE AT OSAS

1. GENERAL

The concept "quality of life" is a relatively new concept which has played a role in Germany only since the middle of the eighties although it was included in the medical literature 10 years earlier in the Anglian American states (ULLRICH 1993, RUPPRECHT 1993). Since the beginning of the nineties it is used almost inflationarily in the everyday language (e.g. pharmaceutical industry, media) (RUPPRECHT 1993).

- The quality of life research has got interesting in the area of the medicine only for some time. Are part of the numerous reasons among others
- the expansion of the health concept on basis of the WHO definition of pure physical aspects on emotional and social
- the increase of not treatable cancer diseasees as well as chronic diseasees this one strengthened research
- to the distinction of different therapy forms
- the risk use tradeoff (relationship of a desired symptom change unwanted condition impairment) in the therapy choice

(BULLINGER 1991, RUPPRECHT 1993).

The "quality of life" serves now as Criterion than at it to judge the success or the failure of medical therapies physically and psychosocially so that a special medical interest in it insists to develop valide measuring instruments into the quality of life recording and to use (RAHM 1993, RUPPRECHT 1993).

The foundation of the EORTC ("European Organization for Research on Treatment of Cancer") was an important step on this way in 1981. In 1993 the first congress found instead of, at the "National Heart, Lung and Blood institutes", which introduced and discussed living quality studies and the problems connected with that. Congress which picked the quality of life out as a central theme also took place in Germany. The congress of the "German Society for Surgery" had the quality of life as a main topic in 1989 (RUPPRECHT 1993).

In the medical research the necessity to investigate the quality of life is recognized by now, this has, however, not gained acceptance in the scientific practice yet. Today, studies to this topic are still very rare (RUPPRECHT 1993).

The main emphases of the quality of life research are on the medical area in the tumorous and the cardiovascular discipline. The first studies to the construct quality of life therefore arose mainly in the tumorous and cardiovascular area (BULLINGER et al. 1991, RUPPRECHT 1993, SCHWARZ 1991, 1994, ULLRICH 1993). Only since some years the concept "quality of life" has increasingly gained meaning also in other medical areas particularly in the sleep medical and neurological.

A general definition of the quality of life nevertheless does not exist, there is only a variety of definition tests which is partly even contradictory (BULLINGER et al. 1991, GLATZER and ZAPF 1984, KATSCHNIG 1994, MEIER-EWERT 1991, NORDEN 1994, RUPPRECHT 1993, STATISTISCHES BUNDESAMT 1994, STOSBERG 1994, ZAPOTOCZKY 1994). A difficulty, which is not overcome to this day, though, a multi-dimensional approach of quality of life is accepted (BULLINGER et al. 1991).

2. QUALITY OF LIFE IN THE SLEEP MEDICINE

In the western societal structures gives a number of patients who are sleep disturbed (e.g. Insomnia, OSAS) and neurological permanently growing too (e.g. Apoplex). The results of the high industrialization, are among others triggering the increase of the societal and social pressure, the growing pressure of competition as well as recognition or performance efforts permanently rising, for this. Before job or flat loss, before financial difficulties or more socially also negative thoughts (among others thoughts of being delivered to such facts helplessly) intensify disregard these negative results as well as the increasing fears resulting from these and change or increase the physiological excitement standard. The emotional loads increased by these, an increasing emotional sensitization as well as its consequences frequently lead to sleep problems and/or to neurological diseasees (among others cerebral ischemias) in turn which strongly affects the quality of life (BÜTTNER 1997, MEYER-EWERT 1988, 1991) or the physical one (BÜTTNER 1997, GÖRTELMEYER 1985, RUPPRECHT 1993).

The influence of sleep disorders on the quality of life can be understood as a multi-dimensional concept which contains three aspects:

- the subjective assessment of the importance of areas of life
- the reaching subjectively or putting into effect aims in life
- conviction which can contribute to the fulfilment of the aims subjectively experienced these --

(BULLINGER 1991, SCHWENKHAGEN et al. 1994).

Already 1967 Monroe compared "good" and "bad" sleepers with each other in his study with physiological and psychological variables.

He found meaningful differences between the two groups at it: the "good" and "bad" sleepers were significantly different in

- the physiological variables
- the psychological variables as well as
- some sleep EEG parameters

(GÖRTELMEYER 1988).

A multi-dimensional model idea also has been used and discussed by Insomnia for the emergence and retention in the research of Insomnia for approx. 15 years. SCHWENKHAGEN et al. examined in 1994 the "day side" of the Insomna with the life satisfaction.

The life satisfaction was train rounding put as a multi-dimensional construct which locked up control convictions and performance assessments in different areas of life.

Clear losses arose in the context of the "bad" ones in all paramenters lifted up in comparison with the "good" sleepers. Experiencing on the day was particularly through

- a less general life satisfaction
- a less subjective performance assessment and
- more negative control convictions
- strongly impaired (SCHWENKHAGEN et al. 1995).

During the day, frequently feel tired, exhausted and sleepy sleep disturbed. Their day atmosphere is impaired considerably (PATEROK 1993).

Mood swings besides increased daytime sleepiness and an increased stress is also described. In the beginning and course of the disease life events charging increased appear particularly in the interhuman area. These still are strengthened or maintained by missing or unsatisfactory coping strategies. The persons affected react to loads braced and show relaxation deficits simultaneously. As a rule, conflicts get internalised. In turn these constant stress lead to the emergence or retention of emotional and/or physical diseasees (SCHWENKHAGEN 1994, 1995).

For the seventh AEP Congress (Association of European Psychiatrists) in 1994 were the correlation of sleepdisorders (particularly Insomnia) and quality of life topic of the satellite symposium. The quality of life was assumed as a multi-dimensional construct also here and the *PCASEE* model designed building on it:

P = Physical problems, sleep, appetite
C = (Cognitive) disorders, concentration, decision ability
A = Affective disorders, fear, depression
S = Social problems, activities of the daily life,
E = Economically/economic social load, financial worries
E = (Ego) personality problem, self acceptance.

The factors of this model interact with each other in a various way and lead to the emergence and retention so from sleep disorders as well as to a reduction of the quality of life (BLAESER-KIEL 1994).

In this study became the connection of the sleep disorders and the quality of life in six European countries which checks the USA and Japan.

It correspondingly was noticed that the sleep disorders affect the quality of life severely particularly by they

- paralyze the day activity
- reduce the fitness
- family and social relations work off
(BLAESER KEEL 1994).

So lead particularly the obstructive Sleep apnea syndrome OSAS (SCHMIDT 1985, GÖRTELMEYER 1985, 1988, BÜTTNER (et al.) 1997, 2002a and b, 2004a, LANGER and SCHULZ 1998, TRUMM et al. 1998, ZEITLHOFER 1998, SANNER et al. 2002, SCHWENKHAGEN et al. 1994, LINDBERG et al.

2006), but also Insomnia and Narkolepsy (BÜTTNER 1997, DIXON et al. 2006), besides physical or physical subsequent diseasees, to restrictions and/or changes frequent also to emotional changes as well as for a reduction of the day state and the quality of life as well as their subjective experience.

The severity degree of the disease and the duration of the therapy having been carried out till now could play a role (OSAS: TRUMM et al. 1998, LANGER and SCHULZ 1998, SANNER et al. 2000, BÜTTNER et al. 2002a and b, 2004a).

There are not greater examinations concerning the quality of life in patients with Sleep-related syndromes (e.g. obstructive Sleep apnea syndrome, Insomnia, Narkolepsy) as well as overview examinations untill now. So at the sleep medical area concerning only examinations there are only some researches regarding the Sleep apnea syndrome, particularly to the *Munich Quality of Life Dimension List* MLDL[3] (BOLITSCHEK 1998, BÜTTNER et al. 1997, 2002a and b, 2004a), to the *Short form 36 of the Health Survey* (BÜTTNER et al. 1997, 2002a and b, 2004a, D'AMBROSIO et al. 1999), to the *Functional Outcomes of Sleep Questionnaire* (WEAVER et al. 1997, BÜTTNER 2005a) and to the *Calgary Sleep Apnea Quality of Life index* (FLEMONS and REIMER 1998, FLEMONS and TSAI 1997, HUI et al. 2000, BÜTTNER 2005b).

---

[3]   MLDL = Münchner Lebensqualitäts-Dimensionen-Liste (english: Munich Quality of Life Dimension List; BULLINGER 1991)

Chapter 7

SUMMARY

In the western social structures the number permanently increases sleep more disturbedly. So already suffer more than 10% of the population from sleep awake disturbances which has to be treated urgently; 800,000 patients suffer under Sleep apnea and 25,000 under Narcolepsy (PETER 1995, PETER et al. 1995). Not diagnosed and untreatedly among others they cause on the one hand frequently subjective sorrow in the persons affected and on the other hand accident danger also increased one due to the increased daytime sleepiness or doziness in the traffic and at work (PETER et al. 1995, GERDESMEYER et al. 1997, RANDERATH et al. 1997, 1998, BÜTTNER et al. 2000a and b).

The Sleep apnea syndrome is an illness happening frequent. Are affected by them 1-5 % of the population (men are concerned by it ten times more than women approx.). A Sleep apnea syndrome is diagnosed if during a 7-hour polygraphic night derivation more than 10 apnea phases/hours appear of more as 10 sec. with a duration.

However, patients with OSAS frequently suffer real symptomatic besides hers at a variety of results among others at an excessive daytime sleepiness (BÜTTNER et al. 2004e), vigilance deficites (BÜTTNER et al. 2003b, BÜTTNER and RÜHLE et al. 2004c) and dysmnesias (BÜTTNER et al. 2003c and d.), during the day, too.

Patients with an obstructive Sleep apnea (YOUNG et al. 1993: 3% of all 30-60-year) suffer, therefore besides their real symptomatic, duration attention frequently reduced at a variety of results, and others at excessive daytime sleepiness and one (GUILLEMINAULT et al. 1978, BRADLEY et al. 1985, PODSZUS et al. 1986, HE et al. 1988, LAMPHERE et al. 1989, ROEHRS et al. 1989, BÉDARD et al. 1991, KRIBBS et al. 1993, MARTIN et al. 1996) (GUILLEMINAULT et al. 1978, BRADLEY et al. 1985, PODSZUS et al. 1986,

HE et al. 1988, LAMPHERE et al. 1989, ROEHRS et al. 1989, BÉDARD et al. 1991, KRIBBS et al. 1993, MARTIN et al. 1996). Nightly Arousals with consecutive sleep fragmentation triggering for this.

This performance restriction influences the persons affected both professionally and in their ability, motor vehicles to lead (FINDLEY et al. 1988a, 1988b, 1989b, 1990, 1991, 1995, MITLER et al. 1988, CASSEL et al. 1991a, 1991b, 1993, 1996, ATS 1994, GERDESMEYER et al. 1997, KRIEGER et al. 1997, RANDERATH et al. 1997, 1998, 2000, WEESS 1997, WEESS et al. 1998a and b, BÜTTNER et al. 2000a and b, BÜTTNER 2001). Accidents or almost accidents are therefore frequently result of this reduced efficiency by falling asleep at the steering wheel. For many patients the symptom tolerance is exceeded with that so that they go in a medical treatment.

Due to these difficulties it seems reasonable to use driving simulators to the Sleep apnea diagnostics since these grasp the duration attention on the one hand globally (FINDLEY et al. 1989, 1990, 1995, GERDESMEYER et al. 1997, RANDERATH et al. 1997, 2000, BÜTTNER et al. 2000a and b, BÜTTNER 2001) and on the other hand also feign the complex performance of driving a car.

George et al. describing the control (tracking) and searching visually over the surroundings after relevant stimuli (visual search) as decisive components of the road performance.

They therefore developed a driving simulator test, which uprised from the divided attention test of Moscowitz et al. (MOSCOWITZ et al. 1977, GEORGE et al. 1996a, 1996b). What is very advisable should replace the initial driving test in the street since it is to handle the driving simulation without risk and with lower effort (GERDESMEYER et al. 1997, RANDERATH et al. 1997, 2000, BÜTTNER et al. 2000a and b, BÜTTNER 2001).

These cognitive deficits can be soothed or lifted under an effective nCPAP therapy. Untreated illnesses can, however, have serious consequences for the persons affected, among others impairments in the weekday, at work and in the traffic.

One can therefore hold tight that sleeplessnesses and/or sleep diseases are complex syndromes summarizing these, be able to impair in his whole personality the person as a whole. You can therefore influence all physical, spiritual and mental processes.

Vigilance can make you reduce the physical and mental efficiency to reduce attention and concentration. You can affect the quality of life, reduce, limit and/or prevent social contacts and competences as well as cause further psychiatric, neurological and organic illnesses.

It is indispensably therefore a detailed sleep diagnostics and if necessary therapy of the till now known sleeplessnesses and/or sleep diseases to bend a therapy resistance forward concerning further physical and mental illnesses and to make an effective medical treatment possible to prevent subsequent illnesses.

REFERENCES

Aldrich, M.S., Automobile Accidents in Patients with Sleep. *Disorders Sleep*, 1989; 12 (6): 483-494.

Aldrich, M.S., Sleep disorders, *Current Opinion in Neurology and Neurosurgery*, 1992; 5: 240-246.

Altmeier M., Bombosch C., Schäfer T., Schläfke M.E., Atmungsantworten auf geringfügige CO_2-Erhöhungen in Abhängigkeit von der Vigilanz beim Menschen, in: Mayer G. (Ed.), *Schlafmedizin in Deutschland 1994*, München: MMV-Verlag, 1995.

American Thoracic Society (ATS), Sleep apnea, sleepiness and driving risk, *Am. J. Respir. Crit. Care Med.*, 1994; 150: 1464-1473.

Andreas S., Hajak G., Natt P., Auge D., Rüther E., Kreuzer H., ST-Streckenveränderungen und Arrhythmien bei obstruktiver Schlafapnoe, *Pneumologie*, 1991; 45 (9): 720-724.

Arruda-Olson A.M., Olson L.J., Nehra A., Somers V.K., Sleep apnea and cardiovascular disease. Implications for understanding erectile dysfunction, *Herz,* 2003; 28 (4): 298-303.

Barbè F., Pericas J., Munoz A., Findley L., Anto JM., Agusti A.G.N., Automobile Accidents in Patients with Sleep Apnea Syndrome, Am J Respir Crit Care Med, 1998; 158: 18-22.

Bassetti C., Aldrich M.S., Sleep apnea in acute cerebrovascular diseases: final report on 128 patients, *Sleep*, 1999; 22 (2): 217-223.

Bates D.W., Schmitt W., Buchwald D., Ware N.C., Lee J., Thoyer E., Kornish R.J., Komaroff A.L., Prevalence of fatigue and chronic fatigue syndrome in a primary care practice. *Arch. Intern. Med.*, 1993; 153: 2759-2765.

Bauer T., Ewig,S., Hasper B., Lüderitz E., Pizzulli L., Schäfer H., Prävalenz der Schlafapnoe bei symptomatischen Patienten mit und ohne koronarer

Herzkrankheit, in: Mayer G. (Ed.), *Schlafmedizin in Deutschland 1994*, München: MMV-Verlag, 1995.

Bäumler G., Mensch und Maschine: Zur Diagnostik der Dauerüberwachungsfähigkeit, *Göttingen: Hogrefe-Verlag*, 1974.

Becker H., Brandenburg U., Conradt R., Köhler U., Peter J.H., Ploch Th., v. Wichert, Einfluß der nCPAP-Therapie auf bradikarde Arrythmien bei Schlafapnoe, *Pneumologie*, 1993; 47 (Suppl. 4): 1993, 706-710.

Becker H., Fus E., Peter,J.H., Schneider H., Stammnitz A., Fortschritte in der nasalen Ventilationstherapie schlafbezogener Atmungsstörungen (SBAS), *Wien Med Wochenschr*, 1994; 144 (Sonderheft): 83-86.

Bèdard M.A., Montplaisir J., Richer F., Malo J., Nocturnal Hypoxemia as a Determinant of Vigilance Impairment in Sleep Apnea Syndrome, *Chest,* 1991; 100: 367-370.

Bèdard M.A., Montplaisir J., Richter F., Malo J., Rouleau I., Persistent neuropsychological deficits and vigilance impairment in sleep apnea syndrome after treatment with continuous positive airway pressure (nCPAP), *J. Clin. Exper. Neuropsychol.*, 1993; 15 (2): 330-341.

Benton A.L., *Der Benton-Test*, Bern/Stuttgart: H. Huber-Verlag, 1974.

Berger M., Hohagen F., Riemann D., Rink K., Schramm E., Weyerer S., Schlafstörungen in der Allgemeinpraxis, in: Engfer A., Hajak G., Rüther E. (Ed.), *Prinzipien und Praxis der Schlafmedizin*, München: MMV-Verlag, 1993.

Beutler T., Haan J., Kognitiv evozierte Potentiale (P300) bei Schlafapnoe-Syndrom, in: Mayer G. (Ed.), *Schlafmedizin in Deutschland 1994*, München: MMV-Verlag, 1995.

Bixler E.O., Vgontzas A.N., Lin H.M., Ten Have T., Leiby B.E., Vela-Bueno A., Kales A., Association of hypertension and sleep-disordered breathing, *Arch. Intern. Med.*, 2000; 160 (15): 2289-2295.

Blaeser-Kiel G., *Zopiclon - Das Hypnotikum für den guten Tag nach der guten Nacht*, Köln: Rhône-Poulenc Pharma GmbH, 1994.

Bolitschek J. et al., Impact of nasal continuous positive airway pressure treatment on quality of life in patients with obstructive sleep apnea, *Eur. Respir. J.,* 1998; 11 (4): 890-894.

Bonnet M.H., Effect of Sleep Disruption on Sleep, Performance and Mood, *Sleep,* 1985; 8 (1): 11-19.

Borck S., Narkolepsie und Narkose, in: Dt. Narkolepsie-Gesellschaft e.V. (Ed.), *Narkose – ein Problem für Narkoleptiker*, Wuppertal: Verlag St. Schmidt, 1995.

Bradley T.D., Rutherford R., Grossman R.F., Lue F., Zamel N., Moldofsky H., Phillipson E.A., Role of daytime hypoxemia in the pathogenesis of right heart failure in the obstructive sleep apnea syndrome, *Am. Rev. Respir. Dis.*, 1985; 131: 835-839.

Braus D.F., Dreßing H., Häfner-Ranabauer W., Hentschel F., Löw L., Schredl M., Kraniale Computertomographische Veränderungen bei Schlafapnoe-Patienten, in: Mayer G. (Ed.), *Schlafmedizin in Deutschland 1994*, München: MMV-Verlag, 1995.

Brickenkamp R., Karl G.A., Geräte zur Messung von Aufmerksamkeit, Konzentration und Vigilanz, in: Brickenkamp R., (Ed.), *Handbuch apperativer Verfahren in der Psychologie*, Göttingen: Hogrefe, 1986, 195-211.

Bullinger M., Ludwig M., v. Steinbüchel N., *Lebensqualität bei kardiovaskulären Erkrankungen*, Göttingen: Hogrefe-Verlag, 1991.

Bullinger M., Kirchberger I., Ware J., Der deutsche SF-36 Health Survey, *Zeitschr. Med. Psychol.*, 1995; 3 (1): 21-36.

Burbach R., Kellner C., Kirchheiner T., Rühle K.-H., Weber U., Der Einfluß von CPAP und BiPAP auf das Herzzeitvolumen bei Patienten mit obstruktiven Schlafapnoe-Syndrom, in: Mayer G. (Ed.), *Schlafmedizin in Deutschland 1994*, München: MMV-Verlag, 1995.

Burmann-Urbanek M., Hörstensmeyer D., Konermann M., Laschewski F., Sanner B., Konstanz der nCPAP-Druckwerte in der Langzeitüberwachung von Patienten mit obstruktiver Schlafapnoe, in: Mayer G. (Ed.), *Schlafmedizin in Deutschland 1994*, München: MMV-Verlag, 1995.

Burwell C.S., Robin E.D., Whaley E.D., Bickelmann A., Extreme Obesity associated with Alveolar Hypoventilation: A Pickwickian Syndrome, *Am. J. Med.*, 1956; 21: 811-818.

Büttner A., Schlafqualität, gesundheitsbezogene *Kontrollüberzeugungen und die Lebensqualität von Narkolepsie-, Insomnie- und OSAS-Patienten, unveröffentlichte Diplomarbeit im Fachbereich Psychologie*, Universität Marburg, 1997.

Büttner A., Randerath W., Rühle K.-H., Der Fahrsimulatortest "carsim" zur Erfassung der Vigilanzminderung von SAS-Patienten. Einfluß verschiedener Faktoren auf die Normwerte, *Pneumologie*, 2000a; 54: 338-344.

Büttner A., Randerath W, Rühle K.-H. Normwerte und Gütekriterien eines interaktiven Fahrsimulators ("carsim"), Somnologie, 2000b; 4: 129-136.

Büttner A., Die Messung der Daueraufmerksamkeit bei Patienten mit Schlafapnoe-Syndrom mittels Fahrsimulator. *Normierung und klinische Überprüfung*, Dissertation, Marburg: Tectum-Verlag, 2001.

Büttner A., Rühle K.-H., Lebensqualität bei obstruktiver Schlafapnoe vor und unter nCPAP, *Pneumologie*, 2002a; 56: 49.

Büttner A., Rühle K.-H., Lebensqualität vor und nach nCPAP – Ein Vergleich mittels MLDL, SF-36, FOSQ und SAQLI, *Somnologie*, 2002b; 6 (Suppl.1): 31.

Büttner A., Rühle K.-H., The Therapeutic Effect of Theophylline on Sustained Attention in Patients with Obstructive Sleep Apnea, *Somnologie*, 2003a; 7: 23-27.

Büttner A., Rühle K.-H., Erfassung von Aufmerksamkeits-Defiziten bei Patienten mit obstruktivem Schlafapnoe-Syndrom mit unterschiedlichen Fahrsimulations-Programmen, *Pneumologie*, 2003b; 57: 722-728.

Büttner A., Alnabary R, Rühle K.-H., Gedächtnisprozesse bei obstruktiver Schlafapnoe vor und unter nCPAP, *Somnologie,* 2003c; 7 (Suppl.1): 62.

Büttner A., Alnabary R, Rühle K.-H., Memory processes of obstructive sleep apnoea patients before and under CPAP therapy, *Abstract b and der IRS + des ISIAN*, 2003d; 104-105.

Büttner A., Rühle K.-H., The Therapeutic Effect of Theophylline on the Sustained Attention in Patients with Obstructive Sleep Apnoea under nCPAP-therapy, *Traffic Injury Prevention,* 2004a; Suppl. CD ICADTS: O-25 (1-6).

Büttner A., Rühle K.-H., Lebensqualität vor und unter nCPAP. Ein Vergleich mittels verschiedener Fragebögen – SWLS, MLDL und SF-36, *Pneumologie* 58; 2004b: 651-659.

Büttner A., Rühle K.-H., Vigilance in case of Sleep Apnea Syndrome, *Abstract b and der ERS + des ISIAN*, 2004c; 215.

Büttner A., Rühle K.-H., Angst und Depression bei OSAS, *Somnologie*, 2004d; 8 (Suppl.1): 47.

Büttner, A., Schimanski Ch., Galetke W., Rühle K.-H., Normierung Epworth Sleepiness Scale (ESS), *Somnologie,* 2004e; 8 (Suppl.1): 63.

Büttner A., Schimanski C., Galetke W., Rühle K.-H., Lebensqualität vor und unter nCPAP-Therapie. Ein Vergleich mittels FOSQ, *Somnologie,* 2005a; 9 (Suppl.1): 31.

Büttner A., Rühle K.-H., Die krankheitsspezifische Lebensqualität vor und unter nCPAP-Therapie bei OSAS mittels SAQLI, *Somnologie*, 2005b; 9 (Suppl.1): 36-37, 52.

Buysse D.Y. et al., The Pittsburgh Sleep Quality Index. a new instrument for psychiatric practice and research, *Psychiatry research* 28 (1984) 193-213.

Cadilhac D.A., Thorpe R.D., Pearce D.C., Barnes M., Rochford P.D., Tarquinio N., Davis S.M., Donnan G.A., Pierce R.J., Sleep disordered breathing in chronic stroke survivors. A study of the long term follow-up of the SCOPES cohort using home based polysomnography, *J. Clin. Neurosci.*, 2005; 12 (6): 632-637.

Carscardon M.J., Dement W.C., Mitler M.M., Roth T., Westbrook P.R., Keenan S., Guidelines for the mutiple sleep latency test (MSLT): a standard measure of sleepiness, *Sleep*, 1986; 9: 519-524.

Cassel W., Stephan S., Ploch T., Peter J.H., Psychologische Aspekte schlafbezogener Atemregulationsstörungen, *Pneumologie*, 1989; 43: 625-629.

Cassel W., Ploch T., Sleep apnea accidents: Health risk for healthy people?, in: Peter J.H., Penzel Th., Podszus T., von Wichert P. (Ed.), *Sleep and Health Risk*, Berlin/Heidelberg/New York: Springer-Verlag, 1991a, 279-285.

Cassel W., Ploch T., Peter H.J., v. Wichert P., Unfallgefahr von Patienten mit nächtlichen Atmungsstörungen, *Pneumologie*, 1991b; 45: 271-275.

Cassel W., Ploch T., Schlafbezogene Atmungsstörungen: Unfallgefahr als psychosozialer Risikofaktor, in: Hecht K., Engfer A., Peter H.J., Poppei M. (Ed.), *Schlaf, Gesundheit, Leistungsfähigkeit,* Berlin/Heidelberg/New York/London/Paris/Tokyo/Hong-Kong/Barcelona/Budapest: Springer-Verlag, 1993, 233-242.

Cassel W., Ploch T., Becker C., Dugnus D., Peter J.H., v. Wichert P., Risk of traffic accidents in patients with sleep-disordered breathing: reduction with nasal CPAP, *Eur. Respir. J.,* 1996; 9: 2606-2611.

Chen I., Scharf S.M., Systemic and myocardial hemodynamics during periodic obstructive apneas in sedated pigs, *J. Appl. Physiol.,* 1998; 84 (4): 1289-1298.

Clarenbach P., Wessendorf T., Sleep and stroke, *Rev. Neurol.* (Paris), 2001; 157 (11 pt 2): 46-52.

Colt H.G., Haas H., Rich G.B., Hypoxemia vs Sleep Fragmentation as Cause of Excessive Daytime Sleepiness in Obstructive Sleep Apnea, *Chest,* 1991; 100: 1542-1548.

Coughlin S.R., Mawdsley L., Mugarza J.A., Calverley P.M., Wilding J.P., Obstructive sleep apnoea is independently associated with an increased prevalence of metabolic syndrome, *Eur. Heart J.,* 2004; 25 (9): 735-741.

Crick F., Mitchison G., The function of dream sleep, *Nature*, 1983; 304: 111-114.

D´Ambrosio C. et al., Quality of life in patients with obstructive sleep apnea. Effect of nasal continuous positive airway pressure–A prospective study, *Chest,* 1999; 115 (1): 123-129.

Damm M., Eckel H.E., Rosenow F., Schneider D., Hypophysenadenome als Ursache eines obstruktiven Schlafapnoe-Syndroms, in: Mayer G. (Ed.), *Schlafmedizin in Deutschland 1994*, München: MMV-Verlag, 1995.

Danner M., Langwieder K., Kritische Analyse der deutschen Unfallstatistik, *Versicherungsmedizin*, 1994; 46 (3): 77-78.

Dement W.C., Kleitman, N., Cyclic variations in EEG during sleep and their relations to eye movements, body motility and dreaming, *Electroencephalography and Clinical Neurophysiology*, 1957; 9: 673-690.

Denzel K., Zimmermann P., Rühle K.-H., Quantitative Untersuchungen zur Erfassung der Tagesmüdigkeit, der Vigilanz und der Aufmerksamkeit vor und nach nCPAP-Therapie bei Schlafapnoesyndrom, *Pneumologie*, 1993; 47: 155-159.

De Olazabal J.R., Miller M.J., Cook W.R., Mithoefer J.C., Disordered breathing and hypoxia during sleep in coronary artery disease, *Chest*, 1982; 82 (5): 548-552.

Dertinger S., Feistel H., Ficker J.H., Hahn G., König H.J., Merkl M., Möller C., Siegfried W., Wolf F., Untersuchungen zur nächtlichen regionalen ZNS-Perfusion beim obstruktiven Schlafapnoe-Syndrom, in: Mayer G. (Ed.), *Schlafmedizin in Deutschland 1994*, München: MMV-Verlag, 1995.

Desaga J.-F., Lämmer C., Schlafapnoe und Prader-Willi-Syndrom (PWS), in: Mayer G. (Ed.), *Schlafmedizin in Deutschland 1994*, München: MMV-Verlag, 1995.

Diaz J., Sempere A.P., Cerebral ischemia: new risk factors, *Cerebrovasc. Dis.*, 2004; 17 (Suppl. 1): 43-50.

Dietze G., Untersuchungen über den Umfang des Bewußtseins bei regelmassig auf einander folgenden Schalleindrücken, *Philosophische Studien*, 1885; 2: 362-393.

Dixon S., Morgan K., Mathers N., Thompson J., Tomeny M., Impact of cognitive behavior therapy on health-related quality of life among adult hypnotic users with chronic insomnia, *Behavioral Sleep Medicine*, 2006; 4 (2): 71-84.

Douglas N.J., Engleman H.M., Effects of CPAP on vigilance and related functions in patients with the sleep apnea/hypopnea syndrome, *Sleep*, 2000; 23 (Suppl. 4): 147-149.

Duchna H.-W., Luckhaupt H., Neumann H., Rasche K., Schultze-Werninghaus G. , Nasale Ventilation bei Patienten mit Schlafapnoe-Syndrom, in: Mayer G. (Ed.), *Schlafmedizin in Deutschland 1994*, München: MMV-Verlag, 1995.

Duchna H.-W., Guilleminault C., Stoohs R.A., Orth M., de Zeeuw J., Schultze-Werninghaus G., Rasche K., Obstruktives Schlafapnoe-Syndrom: Ein kardiovaskulärer Risikofaktor ?, *Z. Kardiol.*, 2001; 90 (8): 568-755.

Duscha Ch., Kotterba S., Rasche K., Widding W., Ereigniskorrelierte Potentiale und neuropsychologische Untersuchungen bei Schlafapnoe-Patienten, in: Mayer G. (Ed.), *Schlafmedizin in Deutschland 1994*, München: MMV-Verlag, 1995.

Ehlenz K., Firle K., Schneider H., Weber K., Peter J.H., Kaffarnik H., v. Wichert P., Reduction of nocturnal diuresis and natriuresis during treatment of obstructive sleep apnea (OSA) with nasal continuous positive air pressure (nCPAP) correlates to cGMP excretion, *Med. Klin.* (Munich), 1991; 86 (6): 294-296, 332.

Engfer A., Meier-Ewert K.H., Diagnose und Therapie von Schlafstörungen unter besonderer Berücksichtigung der Hypersomnien und Parasomnien, in: Engfer A., Rudolf G.A.E. (Ed.), *Schlafstörungen in der Praxis – Diagnostische und therapeutische Aspekte*, Braunschweig/Wiesbaden: F. Vieweg-Verlag, 1990.

Engleman H.M., Cheshire K.E., Deary I.J., Douglas N.J., Daytime sleepiness, cognitive performance and mood after continuous positive airway pressure for thr sleep apnoea/hypopnoea syndrome, *Thorax*, 1993; 48: 911-914.

Engleman H.M., Martin S.E., Deary I.J., Douglas N.J., Effect of continuous positive airway pressure treatment on daytime function in sleep apnoea/hypopnoea syndrome, *Lancet,* 1994; 343 (8897): 572-725.

Faust M., Penzel T., Peter J.H., Podszus T., Schneider H., Weber K., v. Wichert P., Atmung und Schlaf: Schlafbezogene Atmungs-Störungen, in: Berger M. (Ed.), *Handbuch des normalen und gestörten Schlafes,* Berlin/Heidelberg/New York/ London/Paris/Tokyo/Hong-Kong/ Barcelona/Budapest: Springer-Verlag, 1992.

Feuerstein C., Naegele B., Pepin J., Levy P., Fronal lobe-related cognitive functions in patients with sleep apnea syndrome before and after treatment, *Acta Neurologica Belgica*, 1997; 96-107.

Flemons W.W., Reimer M.A., Development of a disease-specific health-related quality of life questionnaire for sleep apnea, *Am. J. Respir. Crit. Care Med.,* 1998; 158: 494-503.

Flemons W.W., Tsai W., Quality of life consequences of sleep-disordered breathing, *J. Allergy Clin. Immunol.,* 1997; 99: 750-756.

Findley L.J., Barth J.T., Powers D.C., Wilhait S.C., Boyd D.G., Suratt P.M., Cognitive Impairment in Patients with Obstructive Sleep Apnea and Associated Hypoxemia, *Chest,* 1986; 90: 686-690.

Findley L.J., Bonnie R.J., Sleep Apnea and Auto Crashes – What is the Doctor to do?, *Chest,* 1988a; 94: 225-227.

Findley L.J., Unverzagt M.E., Suratt P.M., Automobile accidents involving patients with obstructive sleep apnea, *Am. Rev. Respir. Dis.,* 1988b; 138: 337-340.

Findley L.J., Fabrizio M.J., Knight H., Norcross B.B., Laforte A.J., Suratt P.M., Driving simulator performance in patients with sleep apnea, *Am. Rev. Respir. Dis.,* 1989a; 140: 529-530.

Findley L.J., Fabrizio M.J., Thommi G., Suratt P.M., Severity of sleep apnea and automobile crashes, *New England Journal of Medizin*, 1989b; 13: 867-868.

Findley L.J., Weiss J.W., Jabour E.R., Drivers with Untreated Sleep apnea – A Cause of Death and Serious Injury, *Arch. Intern. Med.,* 1991; 151: 1451-1452.

Findley L.J., Automobile driving in sleep apnea, in: Issa F.G., Suratt P.M., Remmers J.E. (Ed.), *Sleep and Respiration*, Wiley-Liss, Inc., 1990, 337-345.

Findley L.J., Weiss W.J., Jabour E.R., Drivers with untreated sleep apnea: a cause of death and serious injury, *Arch Intern. Med.*, 1991; 151: 1451-1452.

Findley L.J., Unverzagt M., Guchu R., Fabrizio M., Buckner J., Suratt P., Vigilance and automobile accidents in patients with sleep apnea or narcolepsy, *Chest*, 1995; 108: 619-624.

Findley L.J., Suratt P.M., Dinges D.F., Time-on-Task Decrements in "Steer Clear" Performance of Patients With Sleep Apnea and Narcolepsy, Sleep, 1999; 22 (6): 804-809.

Findley L.J., Smith C., Hooper J., Dineem M., Suratt P.M.,Treatment with nasal CPAP decreases automobile accidents in patients with sleep apnea, *Am. J. R.espi.r Crit Care Med.*, 2000; 161: 857-859.

Fischer J., Dorow P., Köhler D., Mayer,G., Peter J.H., Podszus T., Raschke F., Rühle K.-H., Schulz, V., Empfehlung zur Diagnostik und Therapie nächtlicher Atmungs- und Kreislaufregulationsstörungen, *Pneumologie*, 1994; 48: 324-327.

Franklin K.A., Cerebral haemodynamics in obstructive sleep apnoea and Cheyne-Stokes respiration, *Sleep Med. Rev.*, 2002; 6 (6): 429-441.

Freitag L., Technische Aspekte der Diagnostik schlafbezogener Atmungsstörungen, in: Konietzko N., Freitag L., Teschler H. (Ed.), *Schlafapnoe,* Berlin/Heidelberg/New York/ London/Paris/Tokyo/Hong-Kong/ Barcelona/ Budapest: Springer-Verlag, 1993.

Fries A., Hetzel C., Pritzel M., Rohmfeld R., Schneider C., Steinberg R., Weeß H.-G., Aufmerksamkeits- und Vigilanzdefizite beim obstruktiven Schlafapnoe-Syndrom und deren Reversibilität nach suffizienter nCPAP-Therapie, in: Mayer G. (Ed.), *Schlafmedizin in Deutschland 1994*, München: MMV-Verlag, 1995.

Fujita S., Conway W., Zorick F., Roth T., Surgical correction of anatomic azbnormalities in obstructive sleep apnea syndrome: uvulopalatopharyngoplasty, *Otolaryngol Head Neck Surg*, 1981; 89 (6): 923-934.

Geibel M., Köhler D., Schönhofer B., Wenzel M., Differenzierung in obstruktives Schlafapnoe-Syndrom und Obesitas Hypoventilationssyndrom durch

Fahrradergometrie, in: Mayer G. (Ed.), *Schlafmedizin in Deutschland 1994*, München: MMV-Verlag, 1995.

Geisler P., Genetische Grundlagen der Narkolepsie, in: Dt. Narkolepsie-Gesellschaft e.V. (Ed.), *Sonderdrucke 1986-1992*, Deutsche Narkolepsie-Gesellschaft, 1993.

George C.F.P., Nickerson P., Hanly P., Miller T., Kryger M., Sleep apnea patients have more automobile accidents (letter), *Lancet*, 1987; 1: 447.

George, C.F.P., Boudreau A.C., Smiley A., Simulated driving performance in patients with obstructive sleep apnea, *Am. J. Respir. Crit. Care Med.*, 1996a; 154: 175-181.

George C.F.P., Boudreau A.C., Smiley A., Comparison of simulated driving perfomance in narcolepsy and sleep apnea patients, *Sleep*, 1996b; 19 (9): 711-717.

George C.F.P., Boudreau A.C., Smiley A., Effects of nasal CPAP on simulated driving performance in patients with obstructive sleep apnea, *Thorax*, 1997; 52: 648-653.

George C.F.P., Smiley A., Sleep Apnea and Automobile Crashes, *Sleep*, 1999; 22 (6): 790-795.

George C.F.P., Vigilance Impairment, Assesment by Driving Simulators, *Sleep*, 2000; 23 (Suppl. 4): 115-118.

Gerdesmeyer C., Randerath W., Rühle K.-H., Zeitliche Abhängigkeit der Fehlerzahl bei Messung der Daueraufmerksamkeit mittels Fahrsimulator vor und nach nCPAP-Therapie bei Schlafapnoesyndrom, *Somnologie*, 1997; 1: 165-170.

Glasz T., *Narkolepsie – Eine Erkrankung der Schlaf-Wach-Regulierung, Facharbeit*, Universität Regensburg, 1996.

Glatzer W., Zapf W. (Ed.), *Lebensqualität in der Bundesrepublik – Objektive Lebensbedingungen und subjektives Wohlbefinde*n, Frankfurt a.M.: Campus-Verlag, 1984.

Glossner-Kleiser G., Herb S., Hetzel J., Hetzel M., Hombach V., Kochs M., Lorch S., Weber J., Auswirkungen der nasalen Überdruckatmungstherapie mit BiPAP und CPAP auf das Herzminutenvolumen und den Lungengefäßwiderstand, in: Mayer G. (Ed.), *Schlafmedizin in Deutschland 1994*, München: MMV-Verlag, 1995a.

Glossner-Kleiser G., Herb S., Hetzel J., Hetzel M., Hombach V., Kochs M., Lorch S., Weber J., Wieshammer S., Zünckel H., Chronotrope Inkompetenz bei obstruktiven Schlafapnoe-Syndrom, in: Mayer G. (Ed.), *Schlafmedizin in Deutschland 1994*, München: MMV-Verlag, 1995b.

Görtelmeyer R., On the Development of a Standardized Sleep Inventory for the Assessment of Sleep, in: Kubicki, St., Herrmann, W.M. (Ed.), *Methods of Sleep Research*, New York: G. Fischer-Verlag, 1985.

Görtelmeyer R., Typologie des Schlafverhaltens. Eine empirische Untersuchung an berufstätigen Personen, in: Wittchen, H.-U. (Ed.), *Beiträge zur klinischen Psychologie und Psychotherapie,* Vol. 4, Regensburg: S. Roderer-Verlag, 1988.

Greenberg G.D., Watson, R.K., Deptula, D., Neuropsychological Dysfunction in Sleep Apnea, *Sleep,* 1987;. 10 (3): 254-262.

Gresele C., Hein H., Eggert F., Beurteilung der Aufmerksamkeitsparameter bei Schlafapnoe-Patienten, *Wien Med. Wochenschr.,* 1996; 146 (13-14): 344-345.

Guilleminault C., Tilkian A., Mitler H.M., The Sleep Apnea Syndromes. *Am. Rev. Med.,* 1976; 27: 465-484.

Guilleminault C., van den Hoed J., Mitler M.M., Clinical overview of the Sleep Apnea Syndromes, in: Guilleminault C., Dement W.C. (Ed.), *Sleep Apnea Syndromes*, New York, Liss., 1978, 1-12.

Guilleminault C., Partinen M., Quera-Salva MA., Hayes B., Dement WC., Nino-Murcia G., Determinants of Daytime Sleepiness in Obstructive Sleep Apnea, *Chest,* 1988; 94: 32-37.

Hajak G., Hauri P.J., Rüther E., Insomnie, in: Berger M. (Ed.), Handbuch des normalen und gestörten *Schlafes,* Berlin/Heidelberg/New York/ London/ Paris/Tokyo/Hong-Kong/Barcelona/Budapest: Springer-Verlag, 1992.

Hajak G., Rüther E., Insomnie - Schlaflosigkeit - Ursachen, Symptomatik und Therapie, Berlin/Heidelberg/New York/ London/Paris/Tokyo/Hong-Kong/ Barcelona/Budapest: Springer-Verlag, 1995.

Hanly P., Sasson Z., Zuberi N., Lunn K., ST-segment depression during sleep in obstructive sleep apnea, *Am. J. Cardiol.,* 1993; 71 (15): 1341-1345.

Harnatt J., Kortikale Aktivierung von Daueraufmerksamkeit, *Psych. Beitr.,* 1975; 17: 188-210.

Harsch I.A., Schahin S.P., Radespiel-Troger M., Weintz O., Jahreiss H., Fuchs F.S., Wiest G.H., Hahn E.G., Lohmann T., Konturek P.C., Ficker J.H., Continuous positive airway pressure treatment rapidly improves insulin sensitivity in patients with obstructive sleep apnea syndrome, *Am. J. Respir. Crit. Care Med.,* 2004; 169 (2): 156-162.

He J., Kryger M.H., Zorick F.J., Conway W., Roth Th., Mortality and apnea index in obstructive sleep apnea. Experience in 385 male patients, *Chest,* 1988; 94: 9-14.

Hein H., Jugert K., Magnussen H., Theophyllin zur Therapie der obstruktiven Schlafapnoe?, *Pneumologie*, 1993; 47: 750-53.

Hein H., Jugert Ch., Kirsten D., Magnussen H., Nikotin zur Therapie der obstruktiven Schlafapnoe ?, in: Mayer G. (Ed.), *Schlafmedizin in Deutschland 1994*, München: MMV-Verlag, 1995a.

Hein H., Jugert Ch., Kirsten D., Magnussen H., Theophyllin zur Therapie der obstruktiven Schlafapnoe ?, in: Mayer G. (Ed.), *Schlafmedizin in Deutschland 1994*, München: MMV-Verlag, 1995b.

Hermann-Maurer E.K. et al., Diagnostisches Inventar nach DSM-III bei Patienten mit schweren Schlafstörungen, *Nervenarzt,* 1990; 61: 28.

Hildebrandt G., Rehmert W., Rutenfranz,J., Twelve- and 24-h rhythms in error frequency of locomotive drivers and the influence of tiredness, *Int. J. Chronobiol.,* 1974; 2: 175-180.

Hildebrandt G., Chronobiologische Grundlagen der Leistungsfähigkeit und Chronohygiene, in: Hildebrandt G. (Ed.), *Biologische Rhythmen und Arbeit*, Wien/New York: Springer-Verlag, 1976, 1-19.

Hochban W., *Das obstruktive Schlafapnoesyndrom – Diagnostik und Therapie unter besonderer Berücksichtigung kraniofazialer Anomalien*, Berlin/Wien: Blackwell Wissenschafts-Verlag, 1995.

Hohagen F., Schönbrunn E., Narkolepsien und andere Formen der Hypersomnie, in: Berger M. (Ed.), *Handbuch des normalen und gestörten Schlafes*, Berlin/Heidelberg/New York/ London/Paris/Tokyo/Hong-Kong/Barcelona/ Budapest: Springer-Verlag, 1992.

Horn J.A., Anderson N.R., Wilkinson R.T., Effects of sleep deprivation on signal detection measures of vigilance. Implications for sleep function, *Sleep*, 1983; 6: 347-358.

Hörstensmeyer D., Laschewski F., Konermann M., Kreuzer I., Sanner B., Sturm A., Obstruktive Schlafapnoe und koronare Herzkrankheit, in: Mayer G. (Ed.), *Schlafmedizin in Deutschland 1994,* München: MMV-Verlag, 1995.

Hennevin E., Hars B., Maho C., Bloch, V., Processing of learned information in paradoxical sleep: Relevanz for memory, *Behavioural Brain Research*, 1995; 69: 125-135.

Hobson, J.A., McCarley R.W., The brain as a dream state generator: An activation – synthesis hypothesis of the dream process, *American Journal of Psychiatry,* 1977; 134: 1335-1348.

Horne J.A., Reyner L.A., Driver sleepiness, *J. Sleep Res.,* 1995; 4 (Suppl. 2): 23-29.

Horstmann S., Hess C.W., Basseti C., Gugger M., Mathis J., Sleepiness-Related Accidents in Sleep Apnea Patients, *Sleep,* 2000; 23 (3): 383-389.

Hui D.S.C., Chan J.K.W., Choy D.K.L., Ko F.W.S., Li Th.S.T., Leung R.C.C., Lai Ch.K.W., Effects of Augmented Continuous Positive Airway Pressure

Education and Support on Compliance and Outcome in a Chinese Population, *Chest*, 2000; 117: 1410-1416.

Ingram F., Henke K.G., Levin H.S., Ingram P.T., Kuna S.T., Sleep Apnea and Vigilance Performance in a Community-Dwelling Older Sample, *Sleep*, 1994; 17 (3): 248-252.

Internationale Klassifikation psychischer Störungen (ICD-10 Kapital V (F)), *Klinisch-diagnostische Leitlinien*, ed.: Dilling H., Mombour W., Schmidt M.H., 2. Aufl., Bern/Göttingen/Toronto/Seattle: H. Huber-Verlag, 1995.

Internationale Klassifikation der Schlafstörungen (ICSD), ed.: Riemann D., Schramm E., Weinheim: Beltz-Verlag, 1995.

James W., *Principles of Psychology*, New York, 1890.

Jenkins J.C., Dallenbach K.M., Obliviscence during sleep and waking, *American Journal of Psychology*, 35, 605-612 (1924).

Jennum P., Hein HO., Suadicani P., Gyntelberg F., Cognitive Function and Snoring, *Sleep*, 1993; 16 (8): 62-64.

Johns M.W., A new method of measuring daytime sleepiness: the Epworth sleepiness scale, *Sleep*, 1991; 14: 540-545.

Johns M.W. et al., Daytime Sleepiness, Snoring and Obstructive Sleep Apnea. The Epworth Sleepiness Scale, *Chest* 1993; 103: 30-36.

Johnson L.C., Sleep Deprivation and Performance, in: Webb W.B. (Ed.), *Biological Rhythms, Sleep and Performance*, New York, Wiley and Sons Ltd, 1982, 111-142.

Jung R., Kuhlo W., Neurophysiological Studies of Abnormal Night Sleep and the Pickwickian Syndrom, *Progr. Brain Res.*, 1965; 18: 140-159.

Kales A., Caldwell A.B., Cadieux R.J., Vela -Bueno A., Ruch L.G., Mayes S.D., Severe Obstructive Sleep Apnea – II: Associated Psychopathology and Psychological Consequences, *J. Chron. Dis.*, 1985; 38 (5): 427-434.

Karni A., Tanne D., Rubenstein B.S., Askenasy J.J.M., Sagi D., Dependence on REM sleep of overnight improvement of a perceptual skill, *Science*, 1994; 265: 679-681.

Katschnig H., Wie läßt sich die Lebensqualität bei psychischen Krankheiten erfassen?, in: Katsching, H., König, P. (Ed.), *Schizophremie und Lebensqualität*, Wien/New York: Springer-Verlag, 1994.

Keller I., Grömminger O., Aufmerksamkeit, in: v. Cramon D. I., Mai N., Ziegler W. (Ed.), *Neuropsychologische Diagnostik*, Weinheim/Basel/Cambridge/New York/Tokio: VCH-Verlag, 1993, 65-90.

Kiely J.L., McNicholas W.T., Cardiovascular risk factors in patients with obstructive sleep apnoea syndrome, *Eur. Respir. J.*, 2000; 16 (1): 128-133.

Kiselak J., Clark M., Pera V., Rosenberg C., Redline, S., The Association between Hpertension and Sleep Apnea in Obese Patients, *Chest,* 1993; 104: 775-780.

Klutmann   I.,   Simon   H.,   Winkels   W.,   Häufigkeit   und Erkennungswahrscheinlichkeit der Schlafapnoe in einer internistischen Krankenhausabteilung, in: Mayer G. (Ed.), *Schlafmedizin in Deutschland 1994,* München: MMV-Verlag, 1995.

Köhler U., Schäfer H., Is obstructive sleep apnea (OSA) a risk factor for myocardial infarction and cardiac arrhythmias in patients with coronary heart disease (CHD)?, *Sleep,* 1996; 19 (4): 283-286.

Konietzko N., Steveling H., Teschler H., Schlafapnoe: Synopsis und Differentialdiagnose, in: Konietzko N., Freitag L., Teschler H. (Ed.), Schlafapnoe, Berlin/Heidelberg/New York/ London/Paris/Tokyo/Hong-Kong/Barcelona/Budapest: Springer-Verlag, 1993a.

Konietzko N., Teschler H., Konservative Thrapie des Schlafapnoesyndroms (SAS), in: Konietzko N., Freitag L., Teschler H. (Ed.), *Schlafapnoe, Berlin/Heidelberg/*New York/ London/Paris/Tokyo/Hong-Kong/ Barcelona/Budapest: Springer-Verlag, 1993b.

Kotterba S., Rasche K., Widdig W., Duscha C., Blombach S., Schultze-Werninghaus G., Malin JP., Neuropsychological investigations and event-related potentials in obstructive sleep apnea syndrome before and during CPAP-therapy, *Journal of the Neurological Sciences,* 1998; 159: 45-50.

Kotterba S., Widdig W., Duscha C., Rasche K., Ereigniskorrelierte Potentiale und neuropsychologische   Untersuchungen   bei   Schlafapnoepatienten. *Pneumologie,* 1997; 51: 712-715.

Kribbs N.B., Getsy J.E., Dinges D.F., Investigation and management of daytime sleepiness in sleep apnea, in: Saunder N.A., Sullivan C.E. (Ed.), *Sleeping and Breathing* 2, New York: M. Dekker Edition, 1993a, 575-604.

Kribbs N.B., Pack A.L., Kline L.R., Getsy J.E., Schuett J.S., Henry J.N., Maislin G., Dinges D.F., Effects of one night without nasal CPAP treatment on sleep and sleepiness in patients with obstructive sleep apnea, *Am. Rev. Despir. Dis.,* 1993b; 147: 1162-1168.

Krieger J., Meslier N., Lebrun T., Levy P., Phillip-Joet F., Sailly J.C., Racineux J.J., Accidents in obstructive sleep apnea patients treated with nasal continuous positive airway pressure. A prospective study, *Chest,* 1997; 112: 1561-1566.

Kryge M.H., Sleep Apnea, *Arch. Intern. Med.,* 1983; 143: 2301-2303.

Kuhn H., Lund R., Zur Compliance der nCPAP-Therapie beim obstruktiven Schlafapnoe-Syndrom, in: Meier-Ewert K.H., Schulz H. (Ed.), *Schlaf und*

Schlafstörungen, Berlin/Heidelberg/New York/ London/Paris/Tokyo/Hong-Kong/Barcelona/Budapest: Springer-Verlag, 1990.

Lamphere J., Roehrs T., Wittig R., Zorick F., Conway W.A., Roth T., Recovery of alertness after CPAP in apnea, *Chest,* 1989; 96: 1364-1367.

Langanke P., Podszus T., Penzel Th., Peter J.H., v. Wichert P., Effekt der der obstruktiven Schlafapnoe auf die Vorlast des rechten Herzens preload of the right heart, *Pneumologie,* 1993; 47 (Suppl. 1): 143-146.

Langer B., Schulz H., Bessert sich die Befindlichkeit von Patienten mit Schlaf-Apnoe-Syndrom unter einer nCPAP-Therapie?, *Somnologie,* 1998; 2 (Suppl. 1): 16.

Langlois P.H., Smolensky M.H., Hsi B.P., Weir F.W., Temporal patterns of reported single-vehicle car and truck accidents in Texas, U.S.A. during 1980-1983, *Chronobiol Int.,* 1985; 2 (2): 131-140.

Lavie L., Sleep apnea syndrome, endothelial dysfunction, and cardiovascular morbidity, *Sleep,* 2004; 27 (6): 1053-1055.

Lavie L., Lavie P., Daily rhythms in plasma levels of homocysteine. *J. Circadian. Rhythms.,* 2004; 2 (1): 5.

Lavie L., Sleep-disordered breathing and cerebrovascular disease: a mechanistic approach. *Neurol. Clin.,* 2005; 23 (4): 1059-1075.

Lavie L., Lavie P., Obstructive sleep apnoea and plasma homocysteine. *Eur. Heart J.,* 2005a; 26 (5): 526-527.

Lavie L., Lavie P., Obstructive sleep apnoea and plasma homocysteine. *Eur. Heart J.,* 2005b; 26 (20): 2210-2211.

Lavie L., Lavie P., Ischemic preconditioning as a possible explanation for the age decline relative mortality in sleep apnea. *Med. Hypotheses*, 2006; 66 (6): 1069-1073.

Lavie P., Sleep Apnea in Industrial Workers, in: Guilleminault C., Lugaresi E. (Ed.), *Sleep-Wake Disorders: Natural history, epidemiology and long-term evolution*, New York: Raven Press, 1983, 127-136.

Lavie P., Silverberg D., Oksenberg A., Hoffstein V., Obstructive sleep apnea and hypertension: from correlative to causative relationship, *J. Clin. Hypertens* (Greenwich), 2001; 3 (5): 296-301.

Lavie P., Pro: Sleep apnea causes cardiovascular disease. *Am. J. Respir. Crit Care Med.,* 2004; 169 (2):147-148.

Leu F.R., Symptomatologie und sozialmedizinische Folgen der Narkolepsie – Katamnestische Untersuchungen an 120 Narkolepsie-Patienten, Dissertation an der Neurologischen Klinik, Technische Universität München, 1992.

Leuenberger U., Jacob F., Swer L., Waravdekar N., Zwillich C., Sinoway L., Surges of muscle sympathetic nerve activity during obstructive apnea are linked to hypoxemia, *J. Appl. Physiol.*, 1995; 79 (2): 581-588.

Levinson P.D., McGarvey S.T., Carisle C., Eveloff S.E., Herbert P.N., Millman R.P., Adiposity and Cardiovascular Risk Factor in Men With Obstructive Sleep Apnea, *Chest,* 1993; 103: 1336-1342.

Levy P., Pepin J.L., Ferretti G., The dynamics of pharyngeal structures in obstructive sleep apnea, *Neurophysiol. Clin.*, 1994; 24 (3): 227-248.

Lindberg E., Berne Ch., Elmasry A., Hedner J., Janson Ch., CPAP treatment of a population-based sample - what are the benefits and the treatment compliance?, *Sleep Med.,* 2006, in print.

Lugaresi E., Cirignotta F., Zucconi M., Mondini S., Lenzi P.L., Coccagna G., Good and poor sleepers: An epidemiological survery of the San Marino population, in: Guilleminault C., Lugaresi E. (Ed.), *Sleep-Wake Disorders: Natural history, epidemioloy and long term evolution,* New York: Raven Press, 1983, 73-85.

Lund R., Diagnose und Therapie von Atemregulationsstörungen, in: Kemper J., Zulley J. (Ed.), *Gestörter Schlaf im Alter,* München: MMV-Verlag, 1994.

Mackworth J.F., Effect of amphetamine on the detectability of signals in a vigilance task, *Canad J. Psychol.,* 1956; 19: 104-110.

Mackworth N., The breakdown of vigilance during prologed visual search, *Q. J. Exp. Psychol.*, 1958; 1: 6-21.

Martin S.E., Engleman H.M., Deary I.J., Douglas N.J., The effect of sleep fragmentation on daytime function, *Am. J. Respir. Crit. Care Med.,* 1996; 153: 1328-1332.

Mathis J., Hess Ch.W., *Das Schlaf-Apnoe-Syndrom, Schweizerische Rundschau Medizin* (Praxis), 1988; 77: 908-919.

Mayer G., Pollmächer T., Meier-Ewert K.H., Schulz H., Zur Einschätzung des Behinderungsgrades bei Narkolepsie, *Gesundheitswesen,* 1993; 55 (7): 337-342.

Meier-Ewert K.H., *Differentialdiagnose abnormer Tagesschläfrigkeit, Schweizerische Rundschau für Medizin,* 1988; 35; 920-925.

Meier-Ewert K.H., Tagesschläfrigkeit. Ursachen, Differentialdiagnose, Therapie, Weinheim: *Edition Medizin,* 1989.

Meier-Ewert K.H, Abnorme Tagesschläfrigkeit – Ansätze einer Typologie, *Therapeutische Umschau,* 1991; 48: 746-750.

Merritt S.L., Sleep-disordered breathing and the association with cardiovascular risk, *Prog. Cardiovasc. Nurs.,* 2004;19 (1): 19-27.

Meslier N., Gagnadoux F., Giraud P., Person C., Ouksel H., Urban T., Racineux J.L., Impaired glucose-insulin metabolism in males with obstructive sleep apnoea syndrome, *Eur. Respir J.,* 2003; 22 (1): 156-160.

Meyer M., Ermüdungsbedingte Fahruntüchtigkeit von Berufskraftfahrern, *Archiv für Kriminologie,* Vol. 185, 1990, 64-79.

Mitler M., Carskadon M., Czeiler C., Dement W., Dinges D., Graeber R., Catastrophes, Sleep and public policy: consensus report, *Sleep,* 1988; 11: 100-109.

Mitler E.A., Mitler M.M., *Der Traum vom guten Schlaf,* München: Arcis-Verlag, 1992.

Mohsenin V., Is sleep apnea a risk factor for stroke? *A critical analysis, Minerva Med.,* 2004; 95 (4): 291-305.

Montplaisir J., Bèdard MA., Richer F., Rouleau I., Neurobehavioral Manifestations in Obstructive Sleep Apnea Syndrome Before and After Treatment with Continuous Positive Airway Pressure, *Sleep,* 1992; 15 (6): 17-19.

Moscowitz H., Burns M., The effects of alcohol and valium, singly and in combination, upon driving-related skills performance. *Proceedings of the 21st Conference of the Association for Automobile Medicine,* Vancouver, BC, 15-17. September 1977, 226-240.

Müller T.H., Paterok B., Hoffmann M.R., Becker-Carus C., Auswirkungen chronischer Schlafrestriktion auf Leistungsfähigkeit, Stimmung und Müdigkeit, *Somnologie,* 1997; 2: 65-73.

Nachtmann A., Stang A., Wang Y.M., Wondzinski E., Thilmann A.F., Association of obstructive sleep apnea and stenotic artery disease in ischemic stroke patients, *Atherosclerosis,* 2003; 169 (2): 301-307.

Naègele B., Thouvard V., Pèpin JL., Lèvy P., Bonnet C., Perret JE., Pellat J., Feuerstein C., Deficits of cognitive Executive Functions in Patients With Sleep Apnea Syndrome, *Sleep,* 1995; 18 (1): 43-52.

Nakamura T., Chin K., Hosokawa R., Takahashi K., Sumi K., Ohi M., Mishima M., Corrected QT dispersion and cardiac sympathetic function in patients with obstructive sleep apnea-hypopnea syndrome, *Chest,* 2004;125 (6): 2107-2114.

Neau J.P., Rev Neurol (Paris), *Vascular disorders and obstructive sleep apnea syndrome* [Article in French], 2001; 157 (11 pt 2): 34-37.

Neau J.P., Paquereau J., Bailbe M., Meurice J.C., Ingrand P., Gil R., Relationship between sleep apnoea syndrome, snoring and headaches, *Cephalalgia,* 2002; 22 (5): 333-339.

Norden G., Sport, Gesundheit und Lebensqualität. Eine Sekundäranalyse österreichischer Daten, in: Weiß, O. (Ed.), *Sport - Gesundheit - Gesundheitskultur*, Wien/Köln/Weimar: Böhlau-Verlag, 1994.

Norman D.A., *Aufmerksamkeit und Gedächtnis*, Weinheim: Beltz-Verlag, 1973.

Obst S., Streß - Schlaf - Pathogene Mechanismen, Dissertation im Fachbereich Philosophie, Universität Zürich, 1989.

Okabe S., Woch G., Kubin L., Role of GABAB receptors in the control of hypoglossal motoneurons in vivo, *Neuroreport,* 1994; 5 (18): 2573-2576.

Olson L.G., King M.T., Hesnsley M.J., Saunders N.A., A Communitiy Study of Snoring and Sleep-Disordered Breathing. Pervalence, Am J Respir Crit Care Med, 1995;152: 711-720.

Oswald W.D., Roth E., *Der Zahlen-Verbindungs-Test (ZVT),* Göttingen/Toronto/Zürich: Hogrefe-Verlag, 1987.

Pakola S.L., Dinges D.F., Pack A.L., Review of regulations and guidelines for commercial and noncommercial drivers with sleep apnea and narcolepsy, *Sleep,* 1995; 18 (9): 787-796.

Parish J.M., Somers V.K., Obstructive sleep apnea and cardiovascular disease, *Mayo Clin. Proc.*, 2004; 79 (8): 1036-1046.

Paterok B., Gruppentherapie bei primären Schlafstörungen: Effektivität eines multifaktoriellen Ansatzes, *Dissertaion der Universität Bielefeld*, Münster/Hamburg: Lit.-Verlag, 1993.

Peter J.H., Fuchs E., Köhler U., Meizner K., Penzel T., Podzus T., Siegrist J., von Wichert P., Studies in the prevalence of sleep apnea activity: Evalution of ambulatory screening results, *Eur. J. Res. Dis.*, 1986; 69 (Suppl. 146): 451-458.

Peter J.H., Podszus T., Das kardiovaskuläre Risiko bei schlafbezogenen Atmungsstörungen, in: Konietzko N., Freitag L., Teschler H. (Ed.), *Schlafapnoe,* Berlin/Heidelberg/New York/ London/Paris/Tokyo/Hong-Kong/Barcelona/Budapest: Springer-Verlag, 1993.

Peter J.H., Obstruktive Schlafapnoe und obstruktives Schnarchen, in: Peter J.H., Köhler D., Knab B., Mayer G., Penzel T., Raschke F., Zulley J. (Ed.), *Weißbuch Schlafmedizin*, Regensburg: S. Roderer-Verlag, 1995, 58-61.

Peter J.H., Köhler D., Knab B., Mayer G., Penzel T., Raschke F., Zulley J., Einleitung, in: Peter J.H., Köhler D., Knab B., Mayer G., Penzel T., Raschke F., Zulley J. (Ed.), *Weißbuch Schlafmedizin,* Regensburg: S. Roderer-Verlag, 1995, 1-2.

Philip P., Mitler M., Sleepiness at the wheel: symptom or behavior ?, *Sleep,* 2000; 23 (Suppl. 4): 119-121.

Phillipson E.A., Remmers J.E., American Thoracic Society, Indications and Standards for Cardiopulmonary Sleep Studies, *Am. Rev. Respir. Dis.,* 1989;139: 559-568.

Poceta J.St., Timms R.M., Jeong D.U., Swui-Ling H., Erman M.K., Mitler M.M., Maintenance of wakefulness test in obstructive sleep apnea syndrome, *Chest,* 1992; 101: 893-897.

Podszus T., Bauer W., Mayer J., Penzel T., Peter J.H., von Wichert P., Sleep apnea and pulmonary hypertension, *Klin. Wochenschr,* 1986; 64: 131-134.

Podszus T., Pulmonaler Hochdruck bei Störungen der respiratorischen Regulation, *Internist* (Berlin), 1988; 29 (10): 681-687.

Posner M.I., Rafal R., Cognitive theories of attention and the rehabilitation of attentional deficits, in: Meier M., Benton A., Diller L. (Ed.), *Neuropsychological Rehabilitation,* Edinburgh: Churchil Livingstone Press, 1987, 182-201.

Posner M.I., Petersen S.E., The attention system of the human brain, *Ann. Rev. Neurosciences,* 1990; 13: 25-42.

Posner M.I., Attention in Cognitive Neuroscience. An Overview, in: Gazzaniga M.S. (Ed.), *The Cognitive Neurosciences,* Cambridge: A Bradford Book, 1995, 615-625.

Prokop O., Prokop L., Ermüdung und Einschlafen am Steuer, *Dtsch. Z. Gerichtl Med.,* 1955; 44: 343-355.

Rahm L., *Psychologische Aspekte von Schlafproblemen,* Bern/Berlin/Frankfurt a.M./New York/Paris/Wien: P. Lang-Verlag, 1994.

Randerath W., Gerdesmeyer C., Ströhlein G., Rühle K.-H., Messung der Vigilanz mittels Fahrsimulator vor und nach nCPAP – Vergleich zweier Simulationsprogramme mit unterschiedlicher Ereignishäufigkeit, *Somnologie,* 1, 1997, 110-114.

Randerath W., Siller C., Gil G., Rühle K.-H., Fahrsimulatortest zur Erfassung der Daueraufmerksamkeit – Untersuchung bei Normalpersonen und bei Patienten mit obstruktiven Schlafapnoe-Syndrom vor und nach Therapie, *Klinik Ambrock Hagen,* 1998.

Randerath W., Gerdesmeyer C., Siller C., Gil G., Sanner B., Rühle K.-H., A test for the determination of sustained attention in patients with obstructive sleep apnea syndrome, *Respiration,* 2000; 67: 526-532.

Rapp G., Aufmerksamkeit und Konzentration, Erklärungsmodelle - Störungen - *Handlungsmöglichkeiten,* Bad Heilbrunn/Obb.: Klinkhardt-Verlag, 1982.

Rauscher H., Popp W., Zwick H., Systemic Hypertension in Snorers With and Without Sleeep Apnea, *Chest,* 1992; 102: 367-371.

Rechtschaffen A., Kales A. *A manual of standardized terminology, techniques and scoring* Institutes system for sleep stages of human subjects. National of Health Publication, No. 204, 1968.

Redline S., Strauss M., Adams N., Winters M., Roebuck T., Spry K., Rosenberg C., Adams K., Neuropsychological function in mild sleep-disordered breathing, *Sleep*, 1997; 20 (2): 160-167.

Roehrs T., Zoricks F., Wittig R., Conway W., Roth T., Predictors of objective level of daytime sleepiness in patients with sleep-related breathing disorders, *Chest,* 1989; 95: 1202-1206.

Roehrs T., Merrion M., Pedrosi B., Stepanski E., Zorick F., Roth T., Neuropsychological Function in Obstructive Sleep Apnea Syndrome (OSAS) Compared to Chronic Pulmonary Disease (COPD), *Sleep*, 1995; 18 (5): 382-388.

Rohmfeld R., Steinberg R., Weeß H.-G., Aufmerksamkeits- und Vigilanzleistung bei Hypersomnien am Beispiel des Schlaf-Apnoe Syndroms, in: Becker-Carus Ch., *Fortschritte der Schlafmedizin – Aktuelle Beiträge zur Insomnieforschug*, Münster/Hamburg: Lit.-Verlag, 1994.

Rollet B., Die integrativen Leistungen des Gehirns und Konzentration: Theoretische Grundlagen und Interventionsprogramme, in: Klauer K.J. (Ed.), *Kognitives Training*, Göttingen: Hogrefe-Verlag, 1993, 257-272.

Rühle K.H., Pneumologische Aspekte der Schlafapnoe, in: Konietzko N., Freitag L., Teschler H. (Ed.), *Schlafapnoe,* Berlin/Heidelberg/New York/ London/Paris/Tokyo/Hong-Kong/Barcelona/Budapest: Springer-Verlag, 1993.

Rupprecht R., Lebensqualität - Theoretische Konzepte und Ansätze zur Operationalisierung, Dissertation der Philosophischen Falkutät I, F.-Alexander-Universität Erlangen-Nürnberg, 1993.

Rützel E., Aufmerksamkeit, in: Hermann T., (Ed.), *Handbuch psychologischer Grundbegriffe*, 1977, 49-58.

Sanner B., Sturm A., Konermann M., Koronare Herzkrankheit bei Patienten mit obstruktiver Schlafapnoe, *Dtsch Med. Wochenschr*, 1996; 121 (30): 931-935.

Sanner B.M., Klewer J., Trumm A. et al., Long-term treatment with continuous positive airway pressure improves quality of life in obstructive sleep apnea syndrome, *Eur. Respir. J.,* 2000; 16 (1): 118-122.

Sanner B.M.,Tepel M., Esser M. et al., Sleep-related breathing disorders impair quality of life in haemodialysis recipients, *Nephrol. Dial Transplant*, 2002; 17 (7): 1260-1265.

Säring W., Aufmerksamkeit, in: v. Cramon D., Zihl J., (Ed.), *Neuropsychologische Rehabilitation*, Berlin: Springer-Verlag, 1988, 157-181.

Schäfer H., Berner S., Ewig S., Hasper E., Tasci S., Lüderitz B., Kardiovaskuläre Morbidität bei Patienten mit obstruktiver Schlafapnoe in Relation zum Schweregrad der respiratorischen Störung, *Dtsch Med. Wochenschr*, 1998; 123 (39): 1127-1133.

Schäfer H., Köhler U., Ewig S., Hasper E., Tasci S., Lüderitz B., Obstructive sleep apnea as a risk marker in coronary artery disease, *Cardiology*, 1999; 92 (2): 79-84.

Schindler L., Schlafstörungen, in: Reinecker H. (Ed.), *Lehrbuch der Klinischen Psychologie – Modelle psychischer Störungen*, Göttingen/Toronto/Zürich: Hogrefe-Verlag, 1994.

Schmidt R.F., Integrative Funktionen des Zentralnervensystems, in: Schmidt R.F., Thews G. (Ed.), *Physiologie des Menschen*, 22. Aufl., Berlin/Heidelberg/New York/Tokio: Springer-Verlag, 1985.

Schmidtke H., *Die Ermüdung*, Bern/Stuttgart: H. Huber-Verlag, 1965.

Schmöttke H., Wiedl K.H., Neuropsychologisches Aufmerksamkeitstraining in der Rehabilitation von Hirnorganikern, in: Klauer K.J. (Ed.), *Kognitives Training*, Göttingen: Hogrefe-Verlag, 1993, 273-298.

Schneider H., Schaub C.D., Chen C.A., Andreoni K.A., Schwartz A.R., Smith P.L., Robotham J.L., O´Donnell C.P., Neural and local effects of hypoxia on cardiovascular responses to obstructive apnea, *J. Appl. Physiol.*, 2000; 88 (3): 1093-1102.

Schwarz R., Die Erfassung von Lebensqualität in der Onkologie, *Dt. Ärzteblatt*, 1991; 88: 5.

Schwarz R., Lebensqualität und Krebs: Onkologische Therapiestudien im Dienste der Überlebensqualität, in: Bellebaum A., Barheier K. (Ed.), *Lebensqualität. Ein Konzept für Praxis und Forschung*, Opladen: Westdeutscher Verlag, 1994.

Schwarzenberger-Kesper F., Becker H., Penzel T., Peter J.H., Weber K., von Wichert P., Die exzessive Einschlafneigung am Tage (EDS) beim Apnoe-Patienten . Diagnostische Bedeutung und Objektivierung mittels Vigilanztest und synchroner EEG-Registrierung am Tage, *Prax. Klin. Pneumol.*, 1987; 41: 401-405.

Schwenkhagen et al., Die Bedeutung des Konzepts der Lebenszufriedenheit: Ein Vergleich guter und schlechter Schläfer; (Kurzfassung) in: Mayer, G. (Ed.), *Schlafmedizin in Deutschland 1994*, München: MMV, 1994.

Schwenkhagen et al., Die Bedeutung des Konzepts der Lebenszufriedenheit: Ein Vergleich guter und schlechter Schläfer, in: Becker-Carus Ch. (Ed.), *Fortschritte der Schlafmedizin – Aktuelle Beiträge zur Insomnie-Forschung*, Münster: Lit.-Verlag, 1995.

Seko Y., Kataoka S., Senoo T., Analysis of driving behaviour under a state of reduced alertness, *Int. J. Vehicle Design* (Spec. Issue on vehicle safety), 1986; 318-330.

Sforza E., Lugaresi E., Daytime sleepiness and nasal continuous positive airway pressure therapy in obstructive sleep apnea syndrome patients: effects of chronic treatment and 1-night therapy withdrawal, *Sleep*, 1995; 18 (3): 195-201.

Shneerson J.M., Smith I.E., In the SF-36 sensitive to sleep disruption ? A study in subjects with sleep apnoea, *J. Sleep Res*, 1995; 4: 183-188.

Shimizu, H., Nakasato, N., Mizoi, K., Yoshimoto, T., Localizing the central sulcus by functional magnetic resonance imaging and magnetoencephalography, *Clin. Neurol. Neurosurg.*, 1997; 99 (4): 235-238.

Silvestrini M., Rizzato B., Placidi F., Baruffaldi R., Bianconi A., Diomedi M., Carotid artery wall thickness in patients with obstructive sleep apnea syndrome, *Stroke*, 2002; 33 (7): 1782-1785.

Smith C., Sleep stages, memory processes and synaptic plasticity, *Behavioural Brain Research,* 1996; 78: 49-56.

Sperling G., The information available in brief visual presentations. *Psychological Monographs,* 1960; 74: 89-95.

Squire L.R., Alvarez P., Retrograde amnesia and memory consolidation: A neurobiological perspektive, *Current Opinion in Neurobiology*, 1995; 5: 169-177.

Statistisches Bundesamt (Ed.), *Datenreport 6 – Zahlen und Fakten über die Bundesrepublik Deutschland 1993/94*, Bonn: Verlag Bonn Aktuell, 1994 (Teil II / B).

Steiner S., Strauer B.E., Funktionale Dynamik des rechten Ventrikels und pulmonare Zirkulation bei obstruktiver Schlafapnoe. Therapeutische Konsequenzen, *Internist* (Berlin), 2004; 45 (10): 1101-1107.

Stephan S., Cassel W., Schwarzenberger-Kesper F., Fett I., Psychological Problems Correlated with Sleep Apnea, in: Peter J.H., Penzel T., Podszus T., v. Wichert P. (Ed.), *Sleep and Health Risk*, Heidelberg: Springer-Verlag, 1991, 167-173.

Steyvers F.J.J.M., Gaillard A.W.K., The effects of sleep deprivation and incentives of human performance, *Psychol. Res.,* 1993; 55: 64-70.

Stooh, R.A., Bingha, L.A., Ito, A., Guilleminaul, C., Demen, W.C., Sleep and Sleep Disordered Breathing in Commercial Long-Haul Truck Drivers, *Chest,* 1995; 107: 1275-1282.

Stooh, R.A., Guilleminault, C., Itoi, A., Dement W.C., Traffic Accidents in Commercial Long-Haul Truck Drivers: The Influence of Sleep-Disordered Breathing and Obesity, *Sleep,* 1994; 17 (7): 619-623.

Stosber, M., Lebensqualität als Ziel und Problem moderner Medizin, in: Bellebaum A., Barheier K. (Ed.), *Lebensqualität. Ein Konzept für Praxis und Forschung, Opladen*: Westdeutscher Verlag, 1994.

Stradlin, J.R., Obstructive sleep apnoea and driving, *BMJ*, 1989; 298: 904-905.

Strauch I., Schlaf: Ätiologie/ Bedingungsanalyse, in: Baumann U., Perrez M. (Ed.), *Klinische Psychologie*, Vol. I, Bern: H. Huber-Verlag, 1990.

Sullivan C.E., Issa F.G., Berthon-Jones M., Eves I., Reversal of obstructive sleep apnea by continuous positive airway pressure applied through the nares, *Lancet,* 1981; 4: 862-865.

Sullivan C.E., Grunstein R.R., Continuous positive airways pressure in sleep-disordered breathing, in: Kryger M.H., Roth T., Dement W.C. (Ed.), *Principles and Practice of Sleep Medicine,* Philadelphia: W.B. Saunders Co., 1989.

Svatikova A., Wolk R., Magera M.J., Shamsuzzaman A.S., Phillips B.G., Somers V.K., Plasma homocysteine in obstructive sleep apnoea, *European Heart Journal,* 2004; 25: 1325-1329.

Svatikova A., Wolk R., Lerman L.O., Juncos L.A., Greene E.L., McConnell J.P., Somers V.K., Oxidative stress in obstructive sleep apnoea, *European Heart Journal,* 2005; 26: 2435-2439.

Telakivi T., Kajaste S., Partinen M., Koskenvuo M., Salmi,T., Kaprio J., Cognitive Function in Middle-aged Snorers and Controls: Role of Excessive Daytime Somnolence and Slep-Related Hypoxic Events, *Sleep,* 1988; 11 (5): 454-462.

Terán-Santos J., Jimènez-Gomez A., Cordero-Guevara J., The Association Between Sleep Apnea And The Risk Of Traffic Accidents, *N. Engl. J. Med.,* 1999; 340: 847-851.

Tilkian A.G., Guilleminault C., Schroeder J.S., Lehrman K.L., Simmons F.B., Dement W.C., Hemodynamics in sleep-induced apnea. Studies during wakefulness and sleep, *Ann. Intern. Med.* 1976; 85 (6): 714-719.

Tilkian A.G., Guilleminault C., Schroeder J.S., Lehrman K.L., Simmons F.B., Dement W.C., Sleep-induced apnea syndrome. Prevalence of cardiac arrhythmias and their reversal after tracheostomy, *Am. J. Med.,* 1977; 63 (3): 348-358.

Trumm A., Sanner B., Klewer J., Burmann-Urbanek M., Zidek W., Der Einfluß einer Langzeit-nCPAP-Therapie auf die Lebensqualität von Patienten mit obstruktiver Schlafapnoe, *Somnologie*, 1998; 2 (Suppl. 1): 16.

Ullrich J., Die Lebensqualität von Ovarialcarcinom-Patientinnen unter Chemotheraphie, Dissertation im Fachbereich Humanmedizin, Universität Marburg, 1993.

Valencia-Flores M., Bliwise D., Guilleminault C., Cilveti R., Clerk A., Cognitive function in patents with sleep apnea after acute nocturnal nasal continous positive airway pressure treatment, *Journal of Clinical and Experimental Neuropsychology*, 1996; 18 (2): 197-210.

Verstreaten E., Cluydts R., Verbraecken J., de Roeck J., Neuropsychological functioning and determinants of morning alertness in patients with sleep apnea syndrom, *Journal of the International Neuropsychological Society*, 1996; 2 (4): 306-314.

v. Kanel R., Dimsdale J.E., Hemostatic alterations in patients with obstructive sleep apnea and the implications for cardiovascular disease, *Chest,* 2003; 124 (5): 1956-1967.

Walsleben J.A., The measurement of daytime wakefulness, *Chest,* 1992; 101: 890-891.

Weaver T.E., Laizner A.M., Evans L.K., Maislin,G., Chugh D.K., Lyon,K., Smith P.L., Schwartz A.R., Redline S., Pack A.I., Dinges D.F., Instrument to measure functional status outcomes for disorders of excessive sleepiness, *Sleep*, 1997; 20 (10): 835-843.

Weeß H.-G., Schläfrigkeit und sozialmedizinisches Risiko. Theorethische Grundlagen, *Arbeitspapier des Schlaflabors Pfalzklinik Landeck*, 30.01.97.

Weeß H.-G., Lund R., Gresele C., Böhning W., Sauter C., Steinberg R., AG Vigilanz der DGSM, Vigilanz, Einschlafneigung, Daueraufmerksamkeit, Müdigkeit, Schläfrigkeit. Die Messung müdigkeitsbezogener Prozesse bei Hypersomnien-Theoretische Grundlage, *Somnologie*, 1998a; 2: 32-34.

Weeß H.-G., Lund R., Gresele C., Böhning W., Sauter C., Steinberg R., Vigilanz, Einschlafneigung, Daueraufmerksamkeit, Müdigkeit, Schläfrigkeit: Die Messung müdigkeitsbezogener Prozesse bei Hypersomnien, *Somnologie,* 1998b; 2: 32-41.

Wilkinson R.T., Interaction of lack of sleep with knowledge of results, repeatet testing and individual differences, *J. Exp. Psychol.,* 1961; 62: 263-271.

Wilson M.A., McNaughton B.L., Reactivation of hippocampal ensemble memories during sleep episodes, *Science,* 1994; 265: 676-679.

Wolk R., Kara T., Somers V.K., Sleep-disordered breathing and cardiovascular disease, *Circulation*, 2003a; 108 (1): 9-12.

Wolk R., Shamsuzzaman A.S., Somers V.K., Obesity, sleep apnea, and hypertension, *Hypertension,* 2003b; 42 (6): 1067-1074.

Wolk R., Somers V.K., Cardiovascular consequences of obstructive sleep apnea, *Clin. Chest Med.*, 2003; 24 (2): 195-205.

Yaggi H., Mohsenin V., Obstructive sleep apnoea and stroke, *Lancet Neurol.*, 2004; 3 (6): 333-42.

Yantis M.A., Identifying depression as a symptom of sleep apnea, *J. Psychosoc. Nurs. Ment. Health Serv.*, 1999; 37 (10): 28-34.

Young T., Palta M., Dempsey J., Skatrud J., Weber St., Badr S., The occurrence of sleep-disordered breathing among middle-aged adults, *The New England Journal of Medicine*, 1993; 328 (17): 1230-1235.

Young T., Blustein J., Finn, L., Palta M., Sleepiness, Driving, Accidents: Sleep-Disordered Breathing and Motor Vehicle Accidents in a Population-Based Sample of Employed Adults, *Sleep,* 1997; 20 (8): 608-613.

Zapotoczky H.G., Psychosoziale Voraussetzungen für Lebensqualität, in: Katschnig H., König P. (Ed.), *Schizophrenie und Lebensqualität,* Wien/New York: Springer-Verlag, 1994.

Zeitlhofer J., Schlafstörungen und Lebensqualität – Epidemiologische Daten aus Österreich, *Somnologie*, 1998; 2 (Suppl. 1): 6.

Zimmer M., DQB1-0602 als genetischer Marker für Narkolepsie, in: Dt. Narkolepsie-Gesellschaft e.V. (Ed.), *Sonderdrucke 1986-1992*, Deutsche Narkolepsie-Gesellschaft, 1993.

Zulley J., Crönlein T., Hell W., Langwieder K., *Einschlafen am Steuer: Hauptursache schwerer Verkehrsunfälle*, Wien Med Wochenschr, 1995; 17/18: 473.

INDEX